The Art and Craft of Literacy Pedagogy

T0174690

In tracing community, and how art and craft can be harnessed to express and manifest communities, this book raises fundamental questions and issues about the nature of literacy in everyday lives. Threaded throughout the contributions is an abiding belief in the expansive and flexible nature of literacy, which might one moment involve photography; in the next, drama; and in the next, invite song coupled with movement. Something happens to literacy when it is seen through multiple modalities of meaning and communication: it moves from a *thing* to a thought and a feeling. Pedagogically, the book offers readers a carousel of places and people to witness literacy with, from young children all the way to grandparents. This opens up a sense of geography and age, proving that literacy really does reside in the centre and corners of our lives. With nine chapters by scholars in Canada, the United Kingdom, and the United States, all researching under the umbrella of the same research study, the collection provides a unique perspective on human and aesthetic communication and shows differences between social groups.

This book was originally published as a special issue of *Pedagogies: An International Journal*.

Jennifer Rowsell is Professor and Canada Research Chair in Multiliteracies at Brock University, St. Catharines, Canada. She has written, co-written, and co-edited 20 books on such wide-ranging topics as family literacy, New Literacy Studies, multimodality, youth and popular culture, digital literacies, ethnography, and multiliteracies. She is the co-editor of the Routledge *Expanding Literacies in Education* book series with Cynthia Lewis, and she is the Department Editor of Digital Literacies for *The Reading Teacher*. Her current research interests include applying multimodal, arts-based practices with youth across schooling and community contexts; expanding research methodologies and theories of literacy for digital, immersive, and game-based research; and longitudinal research with families examining ways of visualizing identities.

The Art and Craft of Literacy Pedagogy

Profiling Community Arts Zone

Edited by
Jennifer Rowsell

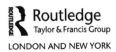

Taylor & Francis Group

LONDON AND NEW YORK

First published 2019
by Routledge
2 Park Square, Milton Park, Abingdon, Oxon, OX14 4RN, UK

and by Routledge
52 Vanderbilt Avenue, New York, NY 10017, USA

First issued in paperback 2020

Routledge is an imprint of the Taylor & Francis Group, an informa business

Introduction, Chapters 1–3, 5–7 © 2019 Taylor & Francis
Chapter 4 © 2017 Abigail Hackett, Kate Pahl and Steve Pool. Originally published as Open Access.
Chapter 8 © 2017 D. McLauchlan

British Library Cataloguing-in-Publication Data
A catalogue record for this book is available from the British Library

ISBN 13: 978-0-367-58380-4 (pbk)
ISBN 13: 978-1-138-38904-5 (hbk)

Typeset in Myriad Pro
by codeMantra

Publisher's Note
The publisher accepts responsibility for any inconsistencies that may have arisen during the conversion of this book from journal articles to book chapters, namely the possible inclusion of journal terminology.

Disclaimer
Every effort has been made to contact copyright holders for their permission to reprint material in this book. The publishers would be grateful to hear from any copyright holder who is not here acknowledged and will undertake to rectify any errors or omissions in future editions of this book.

Contents

CONTENTS

Citation Information

The chapters in this book were originally published in *Pedagogies: An International Journal*, volume 12, issue 1 (January 2017). When citing this material, please use the original page numbering for each article, as follows:

Chapter 6

Embracing the unknown in community arts zone visual arts
Jennifer Rowsell and Peter Vietgen
Pedagogies: An International Journal, volume 12, issue 1 (January 2017) pp. 90–107

Chapter 7

Imperfect/I'm perfect: bodies/embodiment in post-secondary and elementary settings
Kari-Lynn Winters and Mary Code
Pedagogies: An International Journal, volume 12, issue 1 (January 2017) pp. 108–129

Chapter 8

Playlinks: *a theatre-for-young audiences artist-in-the-classroom project*
Debra McLauchlan
Pedagogies: An International Journal, volume 12, issue 1 (January 2017) pp. 130–142

For any permission-related enquiries please visit:
http://www.tandfonline.com/page/help/permissions

Notes on Contributors

Mary Code is a teacher and activist with a passion for creativity in education, 21st century pedagogy, and intersectional feminism. She graduated in 2015 with a master's degree in Education from Brock University, St. Catharines, Canada. She currently teaches English, Drama, and Social Sciences at Fieldstone King's College School, Toronto, Canada.

Daniela Kruel DiGiacomo is a Postdoctoral Researcher in the Graduate School of Education at the University of California Riverside, USA. Her work investigates how to design for more equitable teaching and learning relationships between adults and young people across various lines of difference. She holds a PhD in Learning Sciences and Human Development from the University of Colorado Boulder, USA.

Joyce Duckles is Assistant Professor of Counseling and Human Development at the University of Rochester, USA. She specializes in family studies, community development, informal learning, and participatory research practices. Her current research includes a four-year ethnographic collaborative project on community transformation and a qualitative exploration of the transition of older adults from the Emergency Department to home and the community.

Shelley M. Griffin is Associate Professor of Elementary Music Education at Brock University, St. Catharines, Canada. Her research interests include children's music narratives, pre-service music teacher education, narrative inquiry, Informal faculty mentorship, and collaborative scholarship. She has published in several music education journals and edited books, and has presented at various international conferences. Also, Shelley is an active musician in the Niagara region, performing regularly as a flutist and soprano with Avanti Chamber Singers.

Kris D. Gutiérrez is Carol Liu Professor at the Graduate School of Education, University of California, Berkeley in Learning Sciences and Human Development and in Critical Studies of Race, Class, and Gender. Gutiérrez's work intersects the learning sciences, literacy, educational policy, and qualitative, design-based approaches to inquiry. Gutiérrez is a member of the National Academy of Education and past president of the American Educational Research Association and was appointed by President Obama to the National Board for the Institute of Education Sciences. Gutiérrez's research examines learning in designed environments, with attention to students from nondominant communities and Dual Language Learners. Her work on *Third Spaces* and social design-based experiments seek to leverage students' everyday concepts and practices to ratchet up expansive and equitable forms of learning.

Abigail Hackett is a Research Fellow in the Education and Social Research Institute at Manchester Metropolitan University, UK. Her research focuses on method and theory connected with the lived, embodied everyday experiences of very young children. She is the editor of *Children's Spatialities: Embodiment, Emotion and Agency* (with L. Procter and J. Seymour, 2016).

Courtney Hanny is a graduate of the Warner Graduate School of Education and Human Development at the University of Rochester, USA. She is also a Senior Research Analyst at the SUNY Research Foundation, Buffalo, USA. With a background in art education, literature, and alternative community literacies, her research employs a psychological anthropological approach to social difference, interliteracies, and epistemic justice in learning contexts.

Joanne Larson is the Michael W. Scandling Professor of Education and Associate Director of Research at the Center for Urban Education Success at the University of Rochester, USA. Her ethnographic research examines how language and literacy practices mediate social and power relations in literacy events in schools and communities.

Debra McLauchlan (1951–2016) was a Professor of Drama Education at Brock University, St. Catharines, Canada. Her teaching inspired pre-service teacher education candidates and graduate students in Drama Education with a zest, commitment, and passion for lifelong engagement in the Arts. Her research contributions to the field of education encompassed a wide variety of publications including books, articles, and theatre study guides. A valued colleague, educator, and dear friend of many, she will be sorely missed by all who were blessed to have known her.

Glenys McQueen-Fuentes has just retired after 30 years teaching as an Associate Professor in the Department of Dramatic Arts, Brock University, St. Catharines, Canada. Her areas of expertise and research interests are: physical and international theatre forms, Drama in Education and Applied Theatre and in adapting these areas to explore more effective ways of using movement, drama and music for teaching and learning in all areas of education.

George Moses is Executive Director of North East Area Development and Group 14,621 Community Association, Rochester, USA. He graduated from Monroe Community College, Rochester, USA, where he had the opportunity to represent Community College students across the nation as the VP for Legislative Advocacy for the American Student Association of Community Colleges.

Robert Moses is Director of Economic Development for North East Area Development and Manager of Freedom Market, Rochester, USA.

Kate Pahl is Professor of Arts and Literacy at Manchester Metropolitan University. She is the author of *Materializing Literacies in Communities* (2014). Her current research uses arts based methods and is concerned with feeling 'Odd' in the world of education.

Hoang Pham is a PhD student in the Margaret E. Warner School of Education and Human Development at the University of Rochester, USA. He joined the Freedom Market research group in 2013 and works collaboratively with this community's citizens on this participatory action research project. His PhD research focuses on Southeast Asian American students and their access to college.

Steve Pool trained as a sculptor and now works as a visual artist in multiple media to help people realise ideas, often making physical objects or changing environments. He has an interest in stories, space and co-produced research. He is involved in projects that are concerned with making change with a focus on the role of the artist within society. He has worked on many initiatives including the AHRC Connected Communities program, Creative Partnerships and a number of regeneration projects through area-based renewal programs. In 2010, Steve and fellow artist Kate Genever established. The Poly-technic and work collaboratively to develop arts practice with a focus on social justice. (poly-technic.co.uk). He is now a Phd Candidate at Manchester Metropolitan University.

Jennifer Rowsell is Professor and Canada Research Chair in Multiliteracies at Brock University, St. Catharines, Canada. She has written, co-written, and co-edited 20 books on such wide-ranging topics as family literacy, New Literacy Studies, multimodality, youth and popular culture, digital literacies, ethnography, and multiliteracies. She is the co-editor of the Routledge Expanding Literacies in Education book series with Cynthia Lewis, and she is the Department Editor of Digital Literacies for The Reading Teacher. Her current research interests include applying multimodal, arts-based practices with youth across schooling and community contexts; expanding research methodologies and theories of literacy for digital, immersive, and game-based research; and longitudinal research with families examining ways of visualizing identities.

Peter Vietgen is Associate Professor of Art Education in the Department of Educational Studies at Brock University, St. Catharines, Canada. His research interests include teacher education and the arts; Indigenous education and artistic exploration; museum/gallery museum/gallery education and school partnerships; and social justice and equity studies and the arts. A former Art Consultant/Curriculum Advisor for the Toronto District School Board, he is the current President of the Canadian Society for Education through Art, the national subject association for visual arts education in Canada.

Kari-Lynn Winters is Associate Professor in the Department of Educational Studies at Brock University, St. Catharines, Canada. She is also an award winning Canadian children's author and playwright. Her research interests include multimodal authorship, arts integration, and literacy and children's literature. She is the author of *Youth Claims: Arts, Media, and Critical Literacies in the Lives of Adolescents* (with T. Rogers, M. Perry and A. La Monde, 2014).

Passing through: reflecting on the journey through community arts zone

Jennifer Rowsell

Passing through, passing through.
  Sometimes happy, sometimes blue,
  Glad that I ran into you.
  Tell the people that you saw me passing through.
  Leonard Cohen, 1973

This special issue of *Pedagogies* is devoted to a unique research study that took place across multiple sites in Canada, the United Kingdom, and the United States from September 2013 until May 2015. Built on a belief in community regeneration through arts and literacy initiatives, the international research study reported in the special issue examines different ways that multimodality can be enacted across research contexts. Through the combined expertise of professionals, community members, and arts educators, young people designed and produced texts and improvised on their identities in active, felt ways. Funded by the Canadian government through a Social Sciences and Humanities Research Council Insight Development grant, research featured in this special issue is relational, critical, affective, and semiotic in nature. And, most of all, it is humane.

In the light of its humane qualities, it is worth taking a moment to reflect on our journey since we embarked on the *Community Arts Zone* research study and ended it with this special issue. Just within the research team, the journey has seen changes in our own lives: members of the team have been promoted, moved house, changed universities, and very sadly, one of us has passed away. These are brief, passing references to complex human stories that have taken place behind the scenes over the course of 4 years. Not to mention the world stage with political upheavals, new presidents, and as I wrote this brief introduction, the death of iconic figures like Leonard Cohen. *Life moves on and we pass through it*. But, imprints are made.

The story of *Community Arts Zone* began with the research team's desire to work closely within their respective communities to design and make meaning through modes of expression and representation. At the heart of this special issue is an effort to conduct collaborative, participatory research *with, not on* community members in their idiosyncratic contexts. Researchers from urban and suburban contexts looked inside the lives of people around them through the arts. In this way, we examined diverse ways of knowing through such artistic practices as photography or movement with a broader focus on literacy and cultural and social framings of literacy. Each project, in its own way, applies methodologies like co-production to reimagine how literacy practices in communities are applied and valued. Applying collaborative research methods meant yielding control and ownership of the process, making data collection dynamic, fluid, and at times even messy.

1

Within this special issue, you will encounter toddlers wandering around movable structures; teenagers and children making tableaux; language learners making media texts; community members planning and designing a community mural; teenagers depicting their thoughts, tensions, and convictions in conceptual photographs; first graders making music together; actors working alongside children in schools; and adolescents using drama to consider their bodies and senses of self – what is true across all of the articles is the power of the arts to shake us, affect us, and bind us. And, the arts' capacity to make an imprint on our lives.

Indeed, a driving force of *Community Arts Zone* was to show the possibilities of expansive notions of literacy built around deeper work with modes. The arts and multi-modality furnish wider-angled views of the possibilities for literacy pedagogy and practice. There is a growing awareness that lived literacies have outgrown schooled literacies. By lived literacies we refer to the panoply of ways that people write, design, tweet, read, view, think, compose, snapchat – the list of everyday, lived literacies can go on and on.

Research featured in this special issue brings acts of literacy to life, while correspond-ingly politicizing the frustrating uncertainty and anachronism of formal notions of literacy. Compositions about body image; social studies units put to music; biological processes put to movements; community murals as statements to community members; digital stories about culture and race – these are felt inscriptions performed, viewed, and enacted with what Rancière calls in his work *disensus*. Rancière (2010) maintains that politics is inherently aesthetic in nature and *aesthetics has an inherently political nature*. Rancière argues that the arts and aesthetics move beyond sensible notions to offer transformative action in spaces. There is a politics of sorts that plays out across articles in the special issue: DiGiacomo and Gutiérrez's sensitive and careful rendering of relational equity through multimodal design work built on cultural practices; or, Larson, Hanny, Pham, Moses, and Rutherford's focus on food and healthy eating as the leitmotif of a community designed mural which changed the way community members lived their lives; or, Rowsell and Vietgen's conceptual photographic work that stretched young peoples' capacities to reflect on their lives, afflictions, pleasures, and preoccupations. These topics may strike readers as gentler forms of politics. They make a statement nonetheless.

Participants involved in *Community Arts Zone* were often, literally and metaphorically, brought to life through artistic improvisations. The combined expertise of arts educators with arts professionals amplified sense-making – making multimodal teaching richer, deeper, and bigger in ways that we did not think possible before the research. In a world often characterized by digital communicative practices, research featured in this special issue is digitally light. This is yet another reminder that multimodality cannot be equated with the digital but instead digital domains sit alongside other modal repertoires.

Sustained and profound educational change that is activist and political in nature requires moving beyond more scripted methods and tighter framings to explore com-plexities and entanglements through art-making in communities. Artists know this and recognize the beauty of diverse shapes and frames. Thinking again about the poet and song writer Leonard Cohen who found shapes, light, and frames in his work, as he famously said: "there is a crack, a crack in everything, that's how the light gets in" (Cohen, 1992).

Acknowledgement

We are grateful to the Social Sciences and Humanities Research Council for supporting the research (grant number 430-2013-1025). We are grateful to all of the community members, teachers, students, professionals, Fourgrounds Media, and anyone else who helped to make *Community Arts Zone* such a successful research initiative. We are grateful to all of the reviewers and to *Pedagogies: An International Journal* for making this special issue a reality. A note of thanks as well to Cheryl McLean for providing careful, thoughtful feedback on this introduction. Finally, we are grateful to Jennifer Turner for her meticulous and laborious work on the research – right through to the end of our journey. This special issue is dedicated to the memory of Dr. Debra McLauchlan – a strong advocate for the arts and her Niagara community.

Excerpts from "Anthem" and "Passing Through" by Leonard Cohen. Copyright © Leonard Cohen and Leonard Cohen Stranger Music, Inc, used by permission of The Wylie Agency LLC.

Disclosure statement

No potential conflict of interest was reported by the author.

Funding

We are grateful to the Social Sciences and Humanities Research Council for supporting the research (grant number 430-2013-1025).

References

Cohen, L. (1973). Passing through. *On Live Songs*. The Netherlands: CBS Records.
Cohen, L. (1992). Anthem. *On The Future*. London: Columbia Records.
Rancière, J. (2010). *Dissensus: On politics and aesthetics*. (Translated and edited by S. Corcoran) London, UK: Continuum Press.

Expressing community through freedom market and visual connections

Joanne Larson, Courtney Hanny, Joyce Duckles, Hoang Pham, Robert Moses and George Moses

ABSTRACT

Building on a long-term university/community research partner-ship, this article examines how different ways of conceptualizing, interpreting, and producing murals impacted how an urban com-munity saw itself. Using a participatory action research design, university researchers worked alongside community researchers to ethnographically document the transformation. Findings indi-cate that the mural project constructed pathways for building relationships and community in ways that made neighborhood transformation possible. The mural project embodied this trans-formative goal by providing a space where people gathered with shared attention to talk and to envision how their lives and their community could be different.

Introduction

> Community …. It is an intimate, insider term for the inner city, working class people often apply to themselves and those in their circle of solidarity. (Flower, 2008, p. 22)

How do urban communities transform themselves? Who decides what counts as trans-formation? What systems of knowledge or modes of expression are employed and recognized in initiating and evaluating transformation? These social, historical, political, and epistemological questions became central to the work of community and university activists and researchers working together to improve social and economic futures in one neighborhood. Residents of the Hollywood[1] neighborhood of Rochester grew tired of what they saw as a pattern of "outsiders" coming into their community to "rescue" them. As they expressed it, wave after wave of well-intentioned politicians or university researchers had come to this area of Rochester with a pet program designed to remediate problems identified as needing to be addressed. After a certain amount of time, the project or grant would end without much evidence of change. Any findings or results the research may have generated were not shared with the community, and the neighborhood would be left wondering what was learned, if anything. As a leading community development organization,[2] Northeast Area Development (NEAD) decided to change this dynamic and develop community-driven initiatives using community assets to do the work of transformation themselves. To define community, we, as a collaborative team of university and community researchers, draw upon one resident's comment that, "Community, people have common cultural, living, existence, coexistence" (Interview, January 2015). One community initiative the team began focusing on was the challenge of urban food deserts (Pothukuchi, 2005). Food deserts are geographies common in high-poverty urban areas marked by the absence of access to fresh food within a mile of homes. The Hollywood neighborhood has been identified as such an area. To address this lack of access, NEAD purchased a corner store across the street from their main offices with the explicit goal of transforming the store from a transactional space to a transformative space as part of its mission of economic development, improving education, and improving the quality of life in this neighborhood. This shift toward transformation focused on moving away from simple economic exchange (e.g. store purchases) to relationship building, which emphasized improving how residents viewed their relationship to the community and their role in changing it. Using data from a collaborative ethnography of this effort, now in its sixth year, this article focuses on the residents of this neighborhood, customers who patronize the Freedom Market, the processes of commissioning and creating murals, and the dynamics involved in co-researching these practices. The mural project was sponsored by a Social Sciences and Humanities Research Council of Canada grant under the name Community Arts Zone. Building on the literature about how arts integration impacts community, the research team partnered with this international research group to bring arts and community into dialogic encounters toward new social futures by way of a public art project.

As mentioned briefly above, the Freedom Market started as a community development project intended to address the problem of urban food deserts by transforming a typical urban corner store into a cornerstone of community health and education, a space where relationships were to be built with the goal of transforming how the community viewed itself. A long-term participatory action research (PAR) project was developed, which included these community activists, university professors, graduate students, and, later, local mural artists. The initial object of inquiry for the larger project was on health and nutrition practices, but through a holistic and dialogic approach to data collection and analysis, broad conceptual categories surfaced encompassing a range of emergent and contested ways of knowing. The research team learned that this project was about much more than food once we began the collaborative process of data analysis. It seemed reasonable to the research team to focus on food in a food desert and given that the project began by examining a corner store. However, our collaborative data analysis processes revealed, more importantly, that interactions around food and in the Market were spaces for relationship building. The mural project was an extension of the focus on relationship building as artists, residents, and the research team conceived and installed several murals. It has always been a goal of NEAD to build relationships in each of their initiatives. The mural project embodied this goal by providing a space where people gathered with shared attention to talk and to envision how their lives and their community could be different.

Researching ways of knowing in a PAR context should take account of the institutional discourses or knowledge regimes (Blommaert, 2013) that set the parameters for what constitutes knowledge and how is it valued and recognized. In other words, challenging the parameters set by the academic institutions needs to be part of the project (Nelson, London, & Strobel, 2015). As Flower (2008) recognizes, "'community' stands in sharp relief to the 'university' arriving with its vanload of white, middle-class, educated outsiders, short on savvy, long on good intentions, and comfortably invested in their own set of elite, academic, literate practices" (p. 23). This article presents a close look at the ways in which three discourses (academic, community activist, and artistic) grappled with, and were drawn upon, within the (co)construction of a shared concep-tualization of the murals. "Artistic media," as Percy-Smith and Carney (2010) point out, "are particularly relevant to critical reflexivity because of the multiple interpretations and different ways of seeing that are engendered through the representation or transforma-tion of reality that takes place in the creative process" (Percy-Smith & Carney, 2010, p. 26). This challenge to ways of seeing (interpretation) and to whose voice/knowledge counts (epistemology) came to bear on the development of the murals, their reception, and our research on these processes.

Context for transformation

NEAD is in the Hollywood neighborhood of Rochester which has approximately 6000 residents with area challenges associated with concentrated poverty. NEAD is founded on the seven principles of *nguzo saba*[3] – unity, self-determination, work and responsi-bility, cooperative economics, purpose, creativity, and faith – which guide all the work that they do in this community, and played a key role in collaborative data analysis and the construction of the model of interdependence described below. Following the principle of cooperative economics, NEAD has been working to pull resources that have left the community back in. While the Market project is superficially about food, the work NEAD is doing has always been about economics and relationship building. In addition to the Market, NEAD runs a Children's Defense Fund Freedom School,[4] a pizza parlor, housing development programs, partnerships with local schools on parent engagement, and job development efforts. Recently, it is collaborating with a local university/school educational partnership to reengage students who have dropped out of high school. That program is housed in the Freedom School and prepares students to take the Test for Adult Basic Education.

The work involved in producing the murals we discuss in this article is synonymous with the work NEAD does, specifically the work in the Market. The murals are strategi-cally placed on the outer walls of the Market and main offices across the street. The road between them is a major thoroughfare across town which is used by residents and nonresidents. This is also predominantly a walking neighborhood, with only 40% of residents owning cars. Anyone driving or walking by can see that something transfor-mative is happening and that someone is doing it. As we discuss below, we found that the murals are the embodiment of the transformation of the community and have become part of the walking tour NEAD gives to people interested in their work. In important ways, the murals are pictures of the transformative work of NEAD across all the nodes in our interdependence model.

It was in this context that the idea for murals on the store and the main office emerged during one of our research team meetings. Given that there were two significantly large empty walls at both the Market and the NEAD main office, we imagined together that these spaces could have murals represent the work we do in this community. The research team conceived of the murals as standing for the interaction of word and image. The first mural would be rooted in the mission of *nguzo saba* with the explicit placing of words on stones along the path to freedom. The mission in the second mural would be seen through the sankofa[5] bird which symbolizes reaching back into history to frame the future. What emerged was a set of murals that would be connected through visual messages and intentionally placed locations to represent cultural history, activism, and commitments to the principles of *nguzo zaba* that are deeply rooted in African-American culture in this neighborhood.

Theoretical framework

To make sense of these various interests and concerns that attended the mural component of Freedom Market project, including the academic, community, and artistic discursive traditions, as well as the historical, political, and epistemological concerns that attend any questions of representation, we drew from a range of related theoretical lenses. Theses lenses reflect a dialogical approach to knowledge and identity construction; the recognition that a multimodal (specifically here, the visual) approach to social construction can helpfully dismantle the tendency to rely on strictly textual forms of meaning-making (what might be seen as the dominant modality of the university); and the post-structuralist notion of the rhizomatic nature of knowledge (Deleuze & Guattari, 1987), which eschews a linear or predictable trajectory in favor of a distributed, unpredictable, and generative dissemination of power. A close consideration of how knowledge and meaning were constructed and understood in settings such as the Freedom Market and in the production of the murals required thinking about what, precisely, community identity – with its complex, historical past and positive, possible futures – means to its members, and how that meaning is represented to members and to others. The three discourses mentioned above – academic, community, and artistic – converged in this dialogical space.

   The professors and graduate students who comprise the academic portion of the research team work with the traditions of critical and emancipatory pedagogies that see dialogic interactions (shared spaces in which to speak publicly, deliberate, or voice dissent) as central for bridging or illuminating cultural or ideological divides between variously positioned subjects, hence fostering better understanding and more just ways of being together in communities. The collaborative mural project was particularly illustrative of this dynamic. Shifting away from an emphasis on textuality and individual agency (what might be seen as an academic discourse) toward a more dialogical and multimodal approach to knowledge production opens a way for better understanding the ways that community identity was negotiated in terms of both the development and reception of the mural. As Percy-Smith and Carney (2010) point out, "Visual media facilitate 'knowing' holistically and viscerally without losing the richness and complexity of the experience" (p. 25). Hence the value of murals as testimony to the lived experiences of the community could be foregrounded – as opposed to a more academic analysis of the process or product. Participatory research that employs modalities beyond the strictly textual/linguistic can facilitate participants' practices effort to "claim their collective right to knowledges that are meaningful to their lives" (Licona & Russell, 2013, p. 2). The mural project, both in its collaborative development and its social reception, lent authenticity to representation and dialogical meaning-making across spaces and contexts.

In dialogical approaches to knowledge production and representation, knowledge and meaning are regarded as co-constructed in interactional spaces (i.e. community/ university research teams) by variously positioned interlocutors. This undergirding sensibility, whether it is termed "intersubjectivity," "intertextuality," or "dialogicality" is where cognition happens through interaction. Thinking and concept-building, then, are seen as participatory endeavors (Lave & Wenger, 1991; Nasir & Hand, 2006; Rogoff & Lave, 1984). But participatory endeavors do not equate to shared meanings, and the assumptions that participants are on the same page can work against collaborative efforts (Hanny & O'Connor, 2013; Larson, Webster, & Hopper, 2011). In short, the endeavor to design and produce public murals so that they would serve as an educational tool of sorts, reflecting a complex past and socially conscious future, reflecting local experience and transcultural, diasporadic values, was not only a matter of aesthetics, but a matter of ethics and epistemologies. Licona and Russell (2013) point out that "community literacies" mean "not only the lived, relational, and situated knowledges that circulate in and across communities, but also the ways in which those knowledges are produced and communicated" (p. 1). As Marková (2003) describes such interactional projects, "humans attempt to understand the ways of overcoming the strangeness of cognition of the other person" (p. 33), and "we are not the 'same' in different dialogical relations" (p. 37). Seeing these dialogical tensions as actively impacting the processes, products, and receptions of the mural helped us to understand the richness and complexity of the project as transformative practice.

Lastly, we drew from post-structuralist conceptualizations of knowledge production, identity, and change as dialogical practices. Specifically, we employed the concepts of dialogicality referenced above (Bakhtin, 1981; Marková, 2003) and the rhizomatic structure of interdependence and generativity (Deleuze & Guattari, 1987; Leander & Rowe, 2006) as a theoretical foundation for participatory research. But, as Honeyford (2012) points out, referencing Hall (1997), representation is "a practice, a kind of 'work'" mediated through "material objects and effects" (p. 26). Adopting these perspectives provided a way for us to move between interactional, spatial, and sociocritical frames fluidly, recognizing that they are interdependent and mutually constitutive.

Methodology

The research team consisted of university faculty, doctoral students, and activists from the community development organization that sponsored the Market project and who were also residents of this neighborhood. Together, we collaborated to research the practices of the community, which in turn informed the nature and structure of the project. We followed a PAR (McIntyre, 2008) cycle of data collection–analysis–implementation–collection in iterative cycles to build a local evidence base regarding sociocultural practices. Considering what Kinloch (2009) calls *democratic engagements*, the research team collectively documented the implementation of the mural project in terms residents themselves determined, including the tensions that arose when we tried to speak across different discourses. The research team engaged in qualitative research practices, beginning with teaching community members on the team about how to gather, analyze, and understand their community's practices and to participate in developing solutions to community identified issues.

Our overall data corpus includes more than 6 years' worth of participant observation field notes in and around the Market and during the production of the murals; audio-taped and transcribed interviews with neighborhood residents, Market staff and custo-mers, and artists: audio- and videotaped and transcribed research team meetings; photographs; and surveys. We used a constructivist grounded theory approach for initial coding and analysis (Charmaz, 2014). Members of the research team individually open-coded data sets, then met as a team to develop consensus categories. We worked together to saturate those categories and to build themes, each of which was open to challenge and revision at any point in the process. As a team, we engaged collabora-tively and dialogically with research literature introduced by the academic members and with local expertise in community history, activism, economic and housing develop-ment, and cultural/linguistic practices to produce knowledge about how our initiatives were impacting the community. For this article, we focused on a subset of the larger data corpus of formal interviews with residents, Market staff, and mural artists (~10), participant observation field notes constructed by the research team, and informal interviews with passers-by when the murals were being painted. The research team analyzed these data during our weekly meetings by identifying themes in collaborative discussions.

Developing the model of interdependence

In the larger project, the research team developed the theoretical model of interdependent nodes and networked spaces shown below (Figure 1) – a model that is still open to improvement and development, as new nodes emerge. The research team realized that

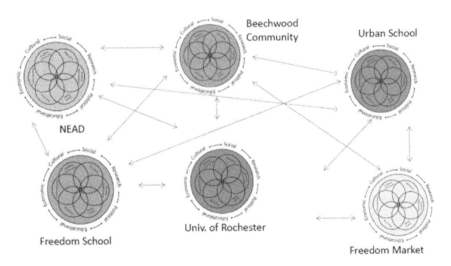

Figure 1. Transformational pathways and developmental trajectories.

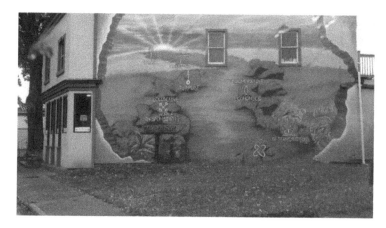

Figure 2. The road to freedom.

it was the same people who worked across various spaces in the neighborhood to achieve the larger transformative goals. This realization led to the concept of nodes, or hubs, within which relationships were developed.

We used the concept of rhizome to understand the travels of sociocultural practices and relationships across the various nodes of interaction. A rhizome is a continuously growing plant that extends shoots and roots at varying intervals. Residents on the research team connected this idea to grassroots organizing, something they are very familiar with, which facilitated the term rhizome becoming part of our shared discourse. Researchers have taken up this concept to account for ways practices spread across spaces and places (Deleuze & Guattari, 1987; Leander & Rowe, 2006). Building on this concept, we found that knowing and meaning making involved a set of practices that were intentionally co-constructed and dialectically enacted across spaces in this community. Within and across each hub (or root), we found six central processes we termed developmental trajectories: building relationships, building community, being family, communicating, belonging, and becoming. We defined them as developmental because of how relationships developed across the nodes and as trajectories because people moved across and through the nodes. Our data demonstrated how, in each space, these trajectories were being intentionally and spontaneously co-constructed by and with community as they moved across and within each node. For example, conversations around the murals focused on history (Africa, slavery), painting (combining colors, conveying a message through visuals), and the problems of poverty, in ways that different ways of knowing were brought together to produce new knowledge about the potential of the neighborhood.

Additionally, we found that transformational pathways situated in the social, cultural, educational, economic, political, and research realms drove and connected these hubs, creating momentum toward sustainable change. People and practices traveled through these pathways to other nodes as well as building new nodes as relationships were developed. We found that the Market was a social space; that it built on cultural practices of food as well as practices of restorative justice (good food for good people); that it created economies through opportunities for the dollars earned in the community to stay in the community; that politics and policies framed the everyday business of the Market and many of the conversations, from school policies to drug laws; that it was an educational space where homework was done, forms were completed, and job training took place; and that it was a research site where community practices and processes of transformation were documented and interpreted. The murals became additional spaces where relationships engendered conversations about possible futures (e.g. the road to freedom) and how the present connects to history (e.g. the sankofa). We found that nurturing these pathways and making them explicit enervated the hubs by creating momentum toward change.

The interactional model is a representation of our finding that people, practices, and discourses emerge and flow across spaces in this community. Part of our work had to consider how people moved across these spaces and how community was developed and sustained. We found that building relationships was a key pathway into community transformation. The mural project served as one entry point to a new transformational pathway, visual imagery, through conversations about the images and the possibilities they represent.

The mural projects

Researchers have defined community art as a "specific, sited-group expression" (Mosher, 2004, p. 530). A mural, as a type of community art, is usually art by an individual in the community or commissioned with the community's input or cognizance of its issues. Mural contents tend to also be driven by humane particularities, such as a community's admitting to concerns of race, class, and spirituality. Some forms of murals are presented as neighborhood celebrations and access to community strengths and assets. The literature has shown that murals can serve as indicators of community identity (Marschall, 1998), community health (Delgado, 1997), community strengths and assets (Delgado & Barton, 1998), democratic art (Mosher, 2004), and to construct neighborhood solidarity (Sieber, Cordeiro, & Ferro, 2012). It was particularly critical for the research team to view the murals from a perspective of community strength and sustainability to better understand the issues at stake for neighborhood residents. Building on these understandings of community art, the mural project engaged local artists to collaborate with community residents, including research team members, to paint spaces where people could gather to talk about the past, present, and future of their community. For the Hollywood neighborhood, the murals provided an interactive space for narratives to emerge about the state of the neighborhood, poverty, and what could be done to transform it. The mural project discussed in this article builds on this experience to understand how dialogic encounters between art, artists, researchers, and community members contributed to community transformation.

This article considers the systematic role that the murals played in bringing the Hollywood community together through analysis of interviews of Freedom Market workers and customers, with the two muralists, and field notes. The first mural was contracted after spending months trying to find an artist. The research team learned that many muralists leave Rochester for winter to paint in the Southern United States. The first mural artist agreed to do the project, even though he did not want community members to do any painting, which was something the research team was committed to given the importance of building relationships in the larger Market project. The artist claimed that it would require much more work than he could handle given that he was now in a wheelchair due to illness. Mostly, he was concerned that he would have to do a lot of repainting and that would take too long; winter was approaching. The research team negotiated various choices regarding the content of the image, settling on one that would represent what we called "the road to freedom." There would be a road that wound through a pastoral landscape, ending in a vibrant sunset that would contain the word "freedom." The seven principles of *nguzo saba* – unity, self-determination, work and responsibility, cooperative economics, purpose, creativity, and faith – would be painted onto stones lining the pathway. Honeyford (2012) points out Hall's (1997) notion that "the visual as a form of *symbolic representation* alludes to the semiotic complexity of visual forms as well as the identity work accomplished through them" (p. 200). The team's goal was that this image would provoke conversations with residents about what their path on the road to freedom might look like.

The team found that the most common question asked when people looked at the road to freedom mural was "what are these words?" Robert Moses and other Market staff consistently responded, "What does it say to you?" One resident said he noticed the connection between the concept of cooperative economics on one of the stones and the practice of extending credit in the store. This noticing prompted a conversation about relationships and supporting one another. Later, Robert reported that this same person donated cash toward the shared pot of money that is used to distribute credit. Another observer noted similarly that the mural revealed what happened in the Market:

> I've seen it here. What the artist did was making it appear as though the store has a hole in it and it shows you what's inside the store and when you look inside the store you see nothing but positive words, positive energy, positive images and the colors stand out. If you look at the actual leaves on the ground, it does, it actually involves and encompasses the whole environment too. It look as though it's a part of the environment vs. here's a building with a painting on it and the painting is a part of the environment, landscape. (Interview, 2015)

Describing the mural as a kind of portal into the positivity inside the Market captured a key feature of how the mural embodies the work NEAD does in the neighborhood. The road to freedom not only leads to transformation but also symbolically leads inside the Market where people support and learn from each other.

The second mural was painted by a woman who was part of the local muralist movement (http://www.wall-therapy.com). This mural focused on collaboration and placemaking. Building on the surroundings of the mural's sociocultural context (this neighborhood, its history, and its possible future), she included figurative, aviary, architectural, and nature-inspired elements when collaborating with community residents, including the research team, to develop the narrative the images would tell. She worked with the research team during team meetings and while painting to develop a vision we are calling "visual connections" that linked the pathways our research had identified to physical spaces throughout the neighborhood using visual images, spoken word, and digital media. This mural was painted on the side of NEAD's main office, directly across the street from the road to freedom mural on Freedom Market. Figure 3 was taken at the

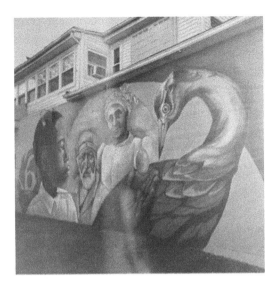

Figure 3. Connecting to history.

formal unveiling of this mural and shows the mural, its relationship to the first mural, and the spoken word poet as he performed to the audience in attendance.

The artist came to several meetings with both small groups and the entire research team. At a team meeting, we decided to create a flyer so that we could pass it out to community members who stopped by to watch the artist painting. "Visual Connections" emerged to tell our story.

We also recognized as a team that we had represented the processes of community transformation through our qualitative data, but the representations had been primarily with words. The artist highlighted the potential of visual imagery:

> It's sometimes hard to connect it visually. Cause, like we were saying, you want it to be open-ended enough that people can see themselves in it. I think sometimes if the visuals are too much ... the same with words. If the words are too much, 'think this' or 'this is what this means,' then people kind of lose interest in it. But if it's beautiful and brings them in, and makes them think about it, then they are going to come with a greater connection to it.

Both the artist and community members agreed that it was valuable having conversations, discussing concepts, and sharing thoughts as the project took shape. Like the reception of the first mural, conversations about the past, the present, and possible futures continued at the second mural. The sankofa image often invoked questions about what it was. These became pedagogical moments for NEAD staff to teach about historical, cultural, and political practices in this community in ways that provoked rethinking how the community might see itself.

Our analysis indicated that the murals impacted the community in three ways: (1) the murals reflected historical expressions about the community, (2) connected to symbols of transformation, and (3) served as spiritual symbols to lead the community to move forward as a whole. Overall, we found that the murals became more than decorative symbols that combined a general message of community belonging and art; they provided an entry point to transformational pathways through the conversations that developed when people stopped to look at them. The murals, as with all the nodes in our model, were spaces where people connected with others and where cross-cultural conversations lead residents and nonresidents to feel connected to each other and to the vision and mission that's been driving the transformation work.

Historical expressions

Throughout the interviews with the muralists and local community members, each of the participants brought up their childhood environments, which motivated them to value positive community resources, such as these murals. The second mural brought into conversation how history impacts the present and the future. Thus, NEAD developed an initiative they called "Visual Connections" that includes the sankofa symbol in all images as an index of reaching back to move forward. The plan is to paint more images across the hubs we have identified in the neighborhood to emphasize interconnectedness and interdependence. Sankofa is a word from the Twi language in Ghana that means to go back and get it. By weaving the sankofa image across these images, history is invoked to understand how to move forward. One community member put it as follows:

> Regarding the mural. It is a history lesson. It is designed based on the history to people who are being enslaved. There are things that they need to do to free themselves from the bond of slavery. There are two bonds: mental bond and physical bond. Obviously, enslaved people are now freed from the physical bond but the emotional bond has been reinforced by the status quo so today it is about how we can break the emotional and intellectual bondage. (Interview, January 2015)

The majority of the individuals who live in the neighborhood are African-American (49%), with some White (35%), and Latinx (16%) (Census, 2016). Given the majority population, African-American cultural history and how the murals, in positive ways, reflected their spiritual enlightenment and battle with oppression was a frequent topic of conversation. For example, all participants discussed that faith (one of the seven principles of *nguzo saba*) was the cornerstone of their well-being and helped them to survive many forms of hardship.

> The road to freedom it requires a collective responsibility of the community. For me, it requires faith and the belief in the father. Definitely you have to have creativity and a purpose behind what you're doing. Cooperative economics has to be taught to individuals to instill a self-determination so that you can unify the neighborhood. That's everything in a nutshell. And, as I look at the sunrise over it, that's the promised land for me. (Interview, June 2015)

As the second mural was being planned we had several discussions about wanting to represent the past and what this meant to participants. A community researcher shared:

> So traditionally when you see pictures of African Americans, it's always the slavery pictures...So the narrative that you get is ... that's why they don't want to remember the past, cause it's like, who wants to remember that? So when you start to get an understanding of well what was in my past, how do I go back to the past to find out what actually happened to bring forward. Remember the bad cause we don't repeat it, but then bring the good things forward.

This community member brought to the meeting a book on his family. He told us his family was one of the original African-American families that settled in Rochester from "Midway" in Florida. He had been given a book with picture of his great, great grandfather on his father's side. He shares his ancestor's first name, and he showed us his image. He reads from the book, telling us that his great, great grandfather was the first property surveyor in Midway. He was surprised that this was a "different narrative" than he had heard – this was different than the slave narrative. He told us the family line from the relatives in this book up to his father, who was, at the time of our conversation, across the street at the corner store frying fish. He explained his history and his family's current identities through his complex family tree.

> So all of those pieces of going back, going back, going back. Then we started looking at them…we got the book and started looking…every last one of them was entrepreneurs. Every last one of them, that's what they did and that's how they survived. So we're like, OK, so it's in the blood. And you don't know, so now that you're aware of what's in the blood, you're able to appropriate all of the energy. 'Cause you were getting the energy because it was going to come through, but once you know what the energy is you get to appropriate all of it, and then it starts to go quantum speed.

The artist said that she was trying to find a way to represent the idea of history:

Artist: I think that was the idea…I was trying to find a way to physically represent that idea of history. And some of that I think was coming from the personal relationship, like the grandfather or grandmother or grandparent or great, great grandparent. I mean, that kind of, was an easier way of describing it than like a universal history. You know what I mean, it like made it specific but could also be something that people relate to. Like, oh that's the past, that's an image of generations. And it might not be your grandfather or you, but it's still like you understand it…versus like trying to speak to this whole neighborhood's history.

George: I get you, I get you, just remember. It can be individual, it can be collective, but for whoever, just remember.

Joyce: That's the only word you really need there, just remember.

We talked about how the image of the sankofa, with the boy being given the egg, represents this passing forward of the past so clearly given that the egg on the bird's back represents the future. It was also decided that we should use faded images of ancestors. The artist requested images, as from the book, rather than picking a specific person to capture the concept of history, the past, and remembering. Conversations that occurred during the painting of the murals offered an entry point for conversations about shared and different histories. Now that the murals are permanent fixtures, these conversations continue as people walk by. There are opportunities to discuss freedom from all perspectives with plenty of space to disagree.

Mural as transformative practice

Many participants pointed out that the murals serve as means to transformative practice. As the first muralist stated:

> I think this painting helps you to see the Hollywood community through a sense of light. It is something positive they can look at and help them strive for some type of success in their life and to overcome the struggles in this neighborhood. It is a beautiful painting to look at it. Something right to look at when you're looking, walking or driving through the neighborhood. Community members had a lot of questions for us when we were painting. We didn't know how big it would be until we started. As the mural progressed, the community embraced it more. It got to the point that people would sit on the porch to enjoy us painting it. They're ingesting the message that the road to freedom. So, that's how we feel about the Hollywood area. This mural helps them to understand. (Interview, February 2015)

Many participants mentioned the murals served a symbolic connection to neighborhood change since the path to freedom must be achieved in different kinds of steps that illustrate adhering to and embracing the symbolic connection between the most intimate home environment to the broad community and cultural values of *nguzo saba*. Others indicated that the murals provided them a space to encourage youth to follow a different pathway, a path away from poverty. Conversations around the murals afforded intergenerational discussions about potential, transformation, and community change. As one community elder put it:

> It says that the neighborhood is ready to change. You have people that is here who are willing and able and trying to help the neighborhood change and the mural definitely does that. It opens your eyes and it opens your mind to things that are going on because a picture is worth a thousand words. (Interview, June 2015)

After talking about the energy of the second mural and moving quantum speed, the executive director of NEAD and member of the research team told us:

> I'm expecting the energy that's created from the sankofa to … actually it's going to (I talk metaphysically sometimes, don't mind me …), it sends a ripple in the universe. I totally expect that. So you've got a major thing you're doing here.

It was also decided that the emphasis should be on the youth, the boy. We recognized as a team that remembering can have both positive and negative connotations, but that we need to remember both. A student researcher commented that in the Black Lives Matter movement, people are so focused on the negative history of black and brown lives, in general, in America:

> … but look at all of the good we've done. And like, the young presence, 'cause it's always been a young presence, young people in the front.

We made connections to the work of the community in these conversations, how much of their work is getting the next-generation ready for this work, for making change. Dialogic encounters around the murals cut across differences in age, race, ethnicity, and language in ways that have potential for transformation.

Moving forward as a community

> Unity here is what we need to have one mind moving forward. We're the people who believe strongly in God ok? Our strong belief and behavior in spiritual ways are our foundations. We had a practice called co-operative economics, self-determination; all of these contribute to our move forward to where we are. We had to be determined but we

also had to be unified. It surrounds our purpose to keep focus to get freedom. We had a bad slavery history, which delayed the practice of our principles. Unity has helped us get to this point. You know, to me, to have the mural right in the middle of the community with people able to view it and coming up with their own interpretation. That's the most important component, to have it here. (Interview, February 2015)

To move forward, participants acknowledged that community residents must recognize and praise their histories as strength. The Visual Connections initiative brings together remembering, moving forward, nourishing, and learning with symbols such as the sankofa bird that index bringing gems of the past to the present. The murals provided an illustration of their historical and cultural practices of celebration and how those practices can shape the future.

The path. It's just an open path as in open minded. If our mind is open, we can accomplish anything. So, as I look at it, all I can see is an open mind headed to the light, to greatness. But, if we're not taught that we're great when we're young, we're not going to head to that. (Interview, June 2015)

The sankofa in the second mural and the extra image that wound around the corner (see Figure 4) emerged as a pivotal image to represent the movement forward across the community. There are plans to continue with murals at the different "hubs" across the community represented in our model. As one community member on the research team stated:

What you're doing is having a tag on all of our buildings. That's how you'll know that's it a part of the movement, cause you're going to see that sankofa bird on the back.

It will be a subtle thing, but consistent. It is conveyed through symbolism. We also decided to add a hashtag to each image – #FreedomSankofa – to build on the connections across multiple spaces and spread the energy and the word.

By engaging the conversation about the murals or to simply gather around them, space exists for interrelation and connection with other residents historically and culturally so that they can collectively move forward. One participant mentioned that having

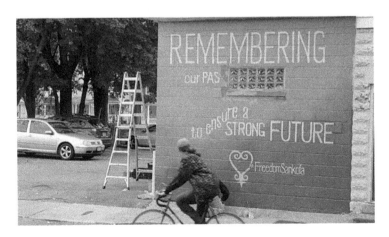

Figure 4. Around the corner.

the murals was enough for people to engage and participate. This realization is a fundamental step for transformation to occur in the neighborhood.

Concluding thoughts

The murals have become spaces for dialogic constructions of pathways to transformation for individuals and for the community as a whole. People gather to look in silence or to talk about what they mean. "Where does the road to freedom lead?" provides an entry point into speaking across difference and into building relationships. Potential for transformation lies in those relationships and how those relationships lead to building community.

Community members on the research team have noted that once we used the frame of reference based on dialogicality – and writing along with rather than writing for – the traditional paternalistic approaches that have grounded many of the change practices in urban communities dissipated. Among our collaborative research group and within the community, the mural project was described as transformational, on the cutting edge of change, and demonstrating new ways of being – of being customers, merchants, and members of a community – of new ways of working with the university. They proposed that this is one of our generation's unique responses to poverty as invested participants intentionally sought to engage individuals in the processes that created these spaces as hubs of change and possibilities, fueled by respect and mutual recognition of difference and potential. We have come to understand the interdependent nodes, specifically the murals, as entry points into intentional pathways to transformation and as creative and positive entry points into the potential of change.

Notes

1. All names are pseudonyms, except Freedom Market, Rochester, and Northeast Area Development (NEAD)
2. NEAD is a not-for-profit neighborhood organization governed by a volunteer board of directors. The volunteers and staff work with city officials and agencies to revitalize and stabilize the Hollywood neighborhood in the northeast quadrant of Rochester, NY. NEAD is organized and operated to improve quality of life through economic development coupled with Housing, Education, Cultural, Recreational, and Social activities. (http://neadRochester.org)
3. The seven principles of *nguzo saba* were developed by Maulana Karenga as the foundation for the African-American celebration of Kwanzaa, which focuses on honoring African-American heritage. http://ibw21.org/vantage-point/the-nguzo-saba-and-kwanzaa-in-a-time-of-crisis/ Accessed on 12/09/16
4. "The *CDF Freedom Schools* program provides summer and after-school enrichment through a model curriculum that supports children and families around five essential components: high quality academic enrichment, parent and family involvement, civic engagement and social action, intergenerational leadership development, and nutrition, health and mental health. In partnership with community based organizations, faith institutions, schools, colleges and universities, the *CDF Freedom Schools* program boosts student motivation to read, generates more positive attitudes toward learning, and connects the needs of children and families to the resources of their communities." http://www.childrensdefense.org/library/data/freedom-schools-fact-sheet.pdf Accessed 12/09/16.
5. Sankofa is a term used by the Akan people of West Africa that means to go back to a community's roots to move forward. Sankofa is represented as a mythic bird that typically has an egg on its back which symbolizes the future. https://www.sankofa.org/mission Accessed 12/09/16

Acknowledgement

The authors wish to gratefully acknowledge the residents of the Beechwood neighborhood of Rochester for their generosity.

Disclosure statement

No potential conflict of interest was reported by the authors.

Funding

This work was partially supported by the Greater Rochester Health Foundation and the Social Sciences and Humanities Research Council of Canada [Grant number 430-2013-1025].

References

Bakhtin, M. 1981. *The dialogic imagination: Four essays* by MM Bakhtin (M. Holquist, ed.; C. Emerson & M. Holquist, trans.).Austin, TX: University of Texas Press.

Blommaert, J. (2013). *Ethnography, superdiversity and linguistic landscapes: Chronicles of complexity.* Tonawanda, NY: Multilingual Matters.

Census (2016). https://www.policymap.com/our-data-directory.html#Census: Decennial Census and American Community Survey (ACS)

Charmaz, K. (2014). *Constructing grounded theory: A practical guide through qualitative analysis* (2nd ed.). London, UK: Sage.

Deleuze, G., & Guattari, F. (1987). *A thousand plateaus: Capitalism and schizophrenia.* Minneapolis, MN: University of Minnesota Press.

Delgado, M. (1997). Strength-based practice with Puerto Rican adolescents: Lessons from a substance abuse prevention project. *Social Work in Education, 19,* 101–112.

Delgado, M., & Barton, K. (1998). Murals in Latino communities: Social indicators of community strength. *Social Work, 43*(4), 346–356. doi:10.1093/sw/43.4.346

Flower, L. (2008). *Community literacy and the rhetoric of public engagement.* Carbondale, IL: SIU Press.

Hall, S. (1997). *Representation: Cultural representations and signifying practices* (Vol. 2). London: Sage.

Hanny, C., & O'Connor, K. (2013). A dialogical approach to conceptualizing resident participation in community organizing. *Mind, Culture, and Activity, 20*(4), 338–357. doi:10.1080/10749039.2012.757322

Honeyford, M. A. (2012). From *aquí* and *allá*: Symbolic convergence in the multimodal literacy practices of adolescent immigrant students. *Journal of Literacy Research, 44*(2), 194–233.

Kinloch, V. (2009). Suspicious spatial distinctions: Literacy research with student across school and community contexts. *Written Communication, 26*(2), 154–182. doi:10.1177/0741088309332899

Larson, J., Webster, S., & Hopper, M. (2011). Community co-authoring: Whose voice remains? *Anthropology and Education Quarterly, 42*(2), 134–153. doi:10.1111/j.1548-1492.2011.01121.x

Lave, J., & Wenger, E. (1991). *Situated learning: Legitimate peripheral participation.* New York, NY: Cambridge University Press.

Leander, K., & Rowe, D. (2006). Mapping literacy spaces in motion: A rhizomatic analysis of a classroom literacy performance. *Reading Research Quarterly, 41*(4), 428–460. doi:10.1598/RRQ.41.4.2

Licona, A. C., & Russell, S. T. (2013). Transdisciplinary and community literacies: Shifting discourses and practices through new paradigms of public scholarship and action-oriented research. *Community Literacy Journal, 8*(1), 1–7. doi:10.1353/clj.2013.0013

Marková, I. (2003). *Dialogicality and self-representations: The dynamics of mind.* Cambridge, UK: Cambridge University Press.

Marschall, S. (1998). A critical investigation into the impact of community mural art. *Transformation, 40,* 55–86.

McIntyre, A. (2008). *Participatory action research.* London, UK: Sage.

Mosher, M. R. (2004). The community mural and democratic art processes. *Review of Radical Political Economics, 36*(4), 528–537. doi:10.1177/0486613404269782

Nasir, N. S., & Hand, V. M. (2006). Exploring sociocultural perspectives on race, culture,and learning. *Review of Educational Research, 76*(4), 449–475. doi:10.3102/00346543076004449

Nelson, I., London, R., & Strobel, K. (2015). Reinventing the role of the university researcher. *Educational Researcher, 44*(1), 17–26. doi:10.3102/0013189X15570387

Percy-Smith, B., & Carney, C. (2010). Using art installations as action research to engage children and communities in evaluating and redesigning city centre spaces. *Educational Action Research, 19*(1), 23–39. doi:10.1080/09650792.2011.547406

Pothukuchi, K. (2005). Attracting supermarkets to inner-city neighborhoods: Economic development outside the box. *Economic Development Quarterly, 19*(3), 232–244. doi:10.1177/0891242404273517

Rogoff, B., & Lave, E. (1984). *Everyday cognition: Its development in social context.* Cambridge, MA: Harvard University Press.

Sieber, T., Cordeiro, G. I., & Ferro, L. (2012). The neighborhood strikes back: Community murals by youth in Boston's communities of color. *City & Society, 24*(3), 263–280. doi:10.1111/ciso.12000

The fluid infusion of musical culture: embodied experiences in a grade one classroom

Shelley M. Griffin

ABSTRACT

Children's daily, embodied music experiences are integral to how children live and function in the world. Growing out of a line of work focusing on the interplay between elementary children's daily experiences of music, both in- and out-of-school and the impact on elementary music education curriculum, this research is nested within the theoretical discourses of experience, children's musical culture, and children's agency. Building upon this work, findings from a two-phase, 6-month inquiry, situated in an urban, Canadian, Grade 1 French Immersion classroom, draw upon the tools of ethnography and narrative inquiry, with the intention of deepening understandings of how informal music-making and sound function in children's lives. Phase one findings highlight: (1) the frequency and spontaneity of children's daily music experiences, both in- and out-of-school, (2) the nature of how music and sound function fluidly in a variety of contexts as integral to children's experience, and (3) the power of musical behaviours in assisting young children to acquire French vocabulary and literacy skills. Important considerations for teacher education include: the necessity of creating space in elementary curriculum to engage children in music-making, integrating and infusing the Arts fluidly across the curriculum, and encouraging children autonomy in their musical engagement.

Introduction

Children embody and embrace music-making experiences in their daily lives, both within informal and formal contexts. Musically rich experiences, both independently and collaboratively, are integral to how children live and function in the world. These experiences provide invaluable enlightenment for conceptualizing elementary school music curriculum and recognizing the place of music education in and across the landscape of curriculum. Emerging from a line of research that focuses on the interplay between children's daily experiences, both in- and out-of-school, and the impact on elementary music education pedagogy and curriculum (Griffin, 2009, 2010, 2011a, 2011b), a new music inquiry developed within the context of the *Community Arts Zone* research. In this article, I focus on the music study, enfolded within the *Community Arts Zone*. As one of eight different projects that is situated across one of four international contexts, the music inquiry sought to examine the interplay between children's in- and out-of-school music experiences. Of particular importance was recognizing the ties between the music research and the broader, overarching goals of *Community Arts Zone*, which were to attend to how: (1) the Arts function as a means to catalyse learning, (2) potential links between the Arts and literacy, and (3) the Arts tie to community. I turn first to offer context between the Arts and literacy and follow this by honouring my own relationship to the research inquiry.

Contextualizing the arts and literacy

The Arts hold an important space in society for understanding the complexities of lives (Halverson & Gibbons, 2009; Honeyford, 2013; Kinlock, 2007). In an increasing digital world, it is valuable to consider the role that the Arts play in contributing towards deepened insight of literacy practices. Through ethnographic research, Kinlock (2007) and Honeyford (2013) signal the need to comprehend the out-of-school experiences of students and how various modes can expand notions of literacy. Halverson and Gibbons (2009) recognize the need to attend to how youth construct and represent identity through engagement with the Arts.

Looking explicitly within the Arts to the context of music, various authors have written about the connections between music-making and language development (Brandt, Gebrian, & Slevc, 2012; Countryman & Gabriel, 2014; Montgomery & Smith, 2014; Walton, 2014; Winters & Griffin, 2014). More specifically, in an ethnomusicological research study focusing on playground language and music-making practices of children aged 5–12, Countryman and Gabriel (2014) found that children engage in multimodal vocal play as they slide along a continuum between speaking and singing. They point out that spontaneous music-making allows for children to experience rhythmic and melodic play which are essential components of language and literacy development. In another example, Montgomery and Smith's (2014) action research study focused on the use of song-based picture books as an integral shared literacy tool between kindergarten-aged children and parents. They determined that the use of song-based picture books provided a space to increase children's fluency with oral language and vocabulary. In our work (Winters & Griffin, 2014), we inquired into how singing and musical experiences provided a platform for lexical acquisition and semantic knowledge. The ethnographic work confirmed that musical involvement allows for children to celebrate language development while building vocabulary. In addition to these ideas regarding music-making and language development, Zeromskaite (2014) draws attention to the importance of music's role in the development of second language learning. After a comprehensive literature review, she concluded that musical training has the potential to improve foreign language pronunciation, receptive phonology, and reading skills. She advocates for increased research in this area so as to deepen understandings regarding music's relationship to second language learning. In summary, all of these researchers believe that children's musical play is a central component to language and literacy development.

Reflexivity: an unfolding story

As I consider my own relationship to this music research study, it is key to honour the unfolding, temporal nature of 20 years that encompass my story as a Canadian music educator, teacher educator, and researcher. My classroom music teaching experience of grades one through nine began in my home province of Prince Edward Island on the east coast of Canada. My desire to improve my teaching practice led me towards graduate studies in Western Canada where I completed both my Masters and PhD degrees, with research focused in music education. For the past 10 years, I have been a teacher educator at Brock University in the Niagara region of Ontario in Central Canada. Experiencing these various Canadian contexts has been informative in providing a breadth and depth of knowledge regarding music education.

I was introduced to the scholarship of Patricia Shehan Campbell (1998) at the conclusion of my Master of Education work (Griffin, 2002) at the University of Alberta, and was inspired by her attention to understand children's informal and formal music-making experiences, with a strong focus of being present to children's perspectives, their voices. Campbell's scholarship resonated with me as her ethnographic work lent attention to studying children over time, developing trust, coming alongside, as the researcher, while listening to what children have to say about their musical experiences.

During my PhD study at the University of Alberta (Griffin, 2007), I also deepened my understandings of narrative inquiry (Clandinin & Connelly, 2000) as a qualitative research method. Under the guidance of Jean Clandinin as one of my doctoral dissertation committee members, I came to conceptualize the role of narrative inquiry research in my doctoral study. My choice to live in these two methodological worlds, ethnography and narrative inquiry, still hold true for my interest to pursue this similar research study again, in a different context, within the *Community Arts Zone* research.

After moving forward from my doctoral dissertation research and the subsequent publications from the study (Griffin, 2009, 2010; Griffin, 2011a, 2011b), I turn now to focus on the current music research inquiry. I begin by contextualizing the three theoretical areas of discourse that lead towards the research purposes and methodological frames. Insights into the life of a particular Grade 1 French Immersion classroom are nested within the rich findings that emerged after spending 6 months in this context, inquiring into the musical lives of a group of young children.

Theoretical underpinnings

The three main theoretical areas that provided the underpinning for conceptualizing the research included *experience* (Barrett & Stauffer, 2009a, 2012b; Clandinin, 2007; Clandinin & Connelly, 2000; Dewey, 1938), *children's musical culture* (Campbell, 2010; Campbell & Wiggins, 2013), and *children's agency* (Ayton, 2012; Corsaro, 2015; Craft, Cremin, Hay, & Clack, 2014; Huf, 2013). Each of these areas is expanded upon so as to provide a central framework that lead toward situating the music inquiry.

Experience

John Dewey (1938) has been one of the most influential theorists in helping educators to conceptualize the importance of experience in relation to education. He believed that there is a dynamic interaction, an intimate and necessary relation between education and personal experience. Thus, experience becomes central to education as there is an organic connection between the two. Dewey cautioned, however, that not all experiences are "genuinely or equally educative" (p. 25). The quality of the experience is central and this impacts how an experience is taken up in future experiences. Dewey identified this notion as the *principle of continuity* which "means that every experience both takes up something from those which have gone before and modifies in some way the quality of those which come after" (p. 34). Thus, a prior experience is influential on future experience. Experience is seen as a moving force and its significance is seen by what it moves towards. Importantly, Dewey viewed experience as social, involving contact and communication with others. He stated that, "There are sources outside an individual which give rise to experience. It is constantly fed from these springs" (p. 40). Therefore, there are factors in the environment outside of the body and mind that shape experience. Dewey urged that educators have the responsibility to shape experience through attending to the conditions of the environment as they recognize "what surroundings are conducive to having experiences that lead to growth" (p. 40).

Clandinin and Connelly (2000) have built upon Dewey's philosophy of experience as a conceptual backdrop to help point educators towards the need to value and study experience through attending to the notion that all experiences have a temporal nature; that is, a past, present, and future. This conceptualization has been central to their thinking about narrative inquiry, both theoretically and methodologically, and the importance of honouring experience through the living, telling, and retelling of storied experience. Clandinin and Connelly affirm, "Experience happens narratively. Narrative inquiry is a form of narrative experience. Therefore, educational experience should be studied narratively" (p. 19). In later writing, Clandinin and Rosiek (2007) explain that narrative inquiry "… begins with an ontology of experience. From this conception of reality as relational, temporal and, continuous, it arrives at a conception of how that reality can be known" (p. 44).

Barrett and Stauffer (2009b, 2012a) have also extended such notions about the relevance of studying experience into the realm of music education research, building a body of scholarship in narrative inquiry in music education. This has been vital work for the field of music education. With a focus on studying musical experience, Barrett and Stauffer (2012b) elaborate: "For narrative inquirers, experience is regarded as both the essence of being and the source of knowing. In other words, how and what we understand ourselves and the world to be are embedded and embodied in experience" (p. 4). Although studying musical experience is a complex matter, it is valued for being rooted in human actions and interactions. It is in such spaces that meaning is created through individual, social, and cultural contexts.

Children's musical culture

Studying musical experience, then, is central to inquiring into children's musical culture. Children embody music-making behaviours in their daily worlds, both independently and collaboratively as they interact with music in their in- and out-of-school places.

While some children may be challenged musically through competition, recitals, or examinations, music is a safe haven for many children; providing a space where they can create and recreate, preserve music and vary it, interact with technological devices, and share music with others. Campbell (2010) has offered seminal work in the area of children's musical culture to help educators and musicologists understand how to tap into the musical thoughts and behaviours of children in order to seek the function of music in their lives. In her ethnographic work, she spent time with young children in various contexts including the schoolyard, school cafeteria, music room, school bus, and a toy store so as to piece together various fragments of children's musical engagement. Campbell stresses the importance of *being* with children, *listening*, and *paying attention* so that music may be understood from their perspectives. Attending to children's voices is integral to understanding the place of music in their daily lives. "Yet musical childhood is largely overlooked and underresearched, particularly with attention to a child-centred approach that gives voice to the children who create their culture, in which music plays a significant role" (Campbell & Wiggins, 2013, p. 5). Importantly, Campbell (2010) has advocated for researching children's musical culture, focusing on children's knowing of music in both in- and out-of-school places. In speaking about the role of music in children's lives, she states,

> They socialize, vent emotions, invent and uphold their rituals of play, and entertain them-selves through music. Their bodies stretch, bend, step, hop, and skip in rhythmic ways, while their melodic voices rise and fall, turn fast and then slow, loud and then soft. Their music can be "seen" and heard in their playful behaviors, some of it a realization of the songs in their heads. It is almost as if children exude music. (p. 4)

Indeed, Campbell reminds us that children are highly sophisticated in their musical actions and the complexities of their musical culture warrant watching and investigating.

Children's agency

Further to the ideas noted regarding musical culture, Dahlberg, Moss, and Pence (1999), Ayton (2012), Craft et al. (2014), and Corsaro (2015) all speak of the importance of providing learning environments that offer contexts for children to have exploration, ownership, and control of their learning through the co-construction of knowledge. Such learning environments are ones that offer children agency in their learning. Agentive learning environments offer possibilities for creative and critical thinking to thrive. Corsaro (2015) explained that children have often been marginalized in society and have been solely seen for what they will become. He articulates,

> ... adults most often view children in a forward-looking way, that is, with an eye to what they will become – future adults with a place in the social order and contributions to make to it. Rarely are they viewed in a way that appreciates what they are – children with ongoing lives, needs, and desires. (p. 6)

Corsaro (2015) speaks of the need for children to be active social agents in the world. This comes with children negotiating, creating, and sharing culture with each other and with adults. The perspective of viewing children as a social construction results from the collaborative actions that children have between one another, as well as the interactions that they have with adults. When children position themselves as agents, they are increasingly able to influence events taking place in their everyday worlds (Ayton, 2012).

Campbell and Wiggins (2013), too, have noted that children are not fully recognized for their agency and are often assigned roles rather than allowing children to discover and create meaning in their learning. In their writing, Campbell and Wiggins noted how essential it is for children to have agency in their learning so as to be able to better understand how children interact with music, both in- and out-of-school, on a daily basis. Craft et al. (2014) also articulate the value of seeing agentive learning both within and beyond school. Freedom, choice, control, and ownership are viewed as pivotal tenants of children's agency as they signal both value and rigour.

Research purpose

Building on the theoretical threads of experience, children's musical culture, and children's agency, the purpose of the research inquiry was to explore the interplay between elementary children's daily experiences of music, both in- and out-of-school and their impact on elementary music education curriculum. The intent was to explore how music and sound functioned in a variety of contexts as integral components of children's daily experiences. Subsequently, it was of interest to be attentive to how children engaged in music-making behaviours across the curriculum to acquire French vocabulary. Accordingly, the research questions guiding the inquiry were: (1) How do children experience music in their daily lives? (2) How do children's musical experiences in their daily lives interplay with their in-school music experiences? and (3) How do children use music to acquire French vocabulary?

Research design: methodological unfoldings

The research inquiry took place in an urban, Southern Ontario, Grade 1 French Immersion classroom. The elementary school (Kindergarten to Grade 8) in which the research took place offered programming in both English and French Immersion. Situated in a mature neighbourhood, the school sat on a 6-acre site that included a large play area which was in close proximity to a treed forest and nearby ravine. Near to the school were many single-family dwellings, as well as university student housing due to the fact that the school was not far from Brock University. Many children frequently walked to school – several were accompanied by a parent or family member. It was common to see parents coming and going, both before and after school. Due to enrolment concerns, since the time that the research was conducted, the school has since closed and was amalgamated with another nearby K–8 English school. A new French Immersion school opened up in the city after the research school closed and a large percentage of those previously enrolled in French Immersion moved to that school. The teaching staff dispersed to various schools within the local school board.

The research school was chosen due to the fact that as the researcher, I had developed a professional relationship and friendship with the teacher who embraces infusing the Arts across the curriculum. I anticipated that her classroom would be an appropriate context to begin to delve into the research questions. We met in June 2013, to begin initial conversations about this possibility. With enthusiasm, she agreed to participate. The teacher indicated that she anticipated that the parents at her school would likely embrace interest and would be eager to become involved. I sensed that there was a sense of community within this school context, a relationship with parents and families beyond the classroom walls. I knew that this research site would fit well within the context of the *Community Arts Zone* project as there was a deep interest in identifying the role that the Arts play out in the broader community. Subsequently, the school principal offered support. After the university ethics and school district approval had been obtained to proceed with the research, all parents of the 22, Grade 1 children (14 girls, 8 boys) agreed to participate, and the field work commenced in January 2014.

The study drew upon the methodological tools of ethnography (Creswell, 2012; Emerson, Fretz, & Shaw, 2011; Jeffrey & Troman, 2004; Van Maanen, 2011) and narrative inquiry (Clandinin & Connelly, 2000; Griffin, 2011c, 2014; Griffin = Beatty, 2012; Kitchen, Ciuffetelli Parker, & Pushor, 2011). These two methodological designs were chosen because as the researcher, I wanted to explore the experiences and behaviours of an entire class of children (ethnography). As time passed and I developed relationships with children, I also desired to come alongside a small group of children, developing a deeper understanding of their music experiences, both in- and out-of-school (narrative inquiry).

The ethnographic perspective was central to exploring the culture-sharing behaviours of a classroom of Grade 1 children. Creswell (2012) describes, "To understand the patterns of a culture-sharing group, the ethnographer typically spends considerable time 'in the field' interviewing, observing, and gathering documents about the group to understand their culture-sharing behaviors, beliefs, and language" (p. 462). This perspective was essential in order to be able to have a deepened, broader understanding of children's daily engagement in the classroom, including observing their interactions with music. Hammersley and Atkinson (2007) indicate that the researcher participates,

> ... in people's daily lives for an extended period of time, watching what happens, listening to what is said, and/or asking questions through informal and formal interviews, collecting documents, and artefacts – in fact, gathering whatever data are available to throw light on the issues that are the emerging focus of inquiry. (p. 3)

Emerson et al. (2011) clarify that the ethnographic perspective ties together two distinct activities: first, spending time in a social setting getting to know the people in the context and second, writing down, in systematic ways, what is observed and experienced in that context.

As was highlighted earlier in the theoretical underpinnings, the study of experience, through the lens of narrative inquiry, was also central to the research inquiry. As a relational form of inquiry, narrative inquiry becomes the way to represent and understand the living and telling of experiences. Clandinin and Connelly (2000) describe that narrative is the best way to represent and understand experience. "Experience is what we study, and we study it narratively because narrative thinking is a key form of experience and a key way of writing and thinking about it" (p. 18). As the researcher, narrative inquiry became the central way for me to live alongside children, developing a relationship of trust while attending to their narratives of experience about their daily musical engagement and musical interactions.

Research phases

The methodological combination of ethnography and narrative inquiry allowed me to create a study involving two phases, over a period of 6 months (January–June 2014). The following chart indicates the timeframe and focus for each phase, as well as the data-gathering tools utilized throughout the research process.

Phase I	Phase II
In-School	Out-of-School
Timeframe • Entire 6-month period	**Timeframe** • Commenced at beginning of fifth month
Focus • Grade 1 in-school music experiences: regular classroom, music classroom, other regular school activities (e.g., recess, lunch, outdoor play)	**Focus** • Six children's out-of-school music experiences: listening to music, family involvement in music, attending musical performances, private music lessons, practice of music outside of school
Data Gathering Tools • Participant observation • Fieldnotes • Informal conversations • Conversations, emails, texts with Gr. 1 teacher • Individual digitally recorded student interviews • Capturing photographic images and video of school life and musical activity • Conversing with parents • *Community Arts Zone* Team talk – meetings and research blog	**Data Gathering Tools** • Same as Phase I plus: • Individual student journals • Conversations and digitally recorded interviews with the families of six children • Teacher interview at conclusion of project

Figure 1. Research Phases.

The first research phase lasted the entire duration of the project. During this time, I investigated the school musical culture of the Grade 1 classroom of children as I observed the daily occurrences in their regular classroom, their music classroom, and during regular school activities (e.g. recess, lunch). All of these contexts were necessary since each provided a space whereby children engaged in music-making. Each week, I spent a full day in the classroom as I watched the children and also was a participant observer in their classroom. With my laptop set up on a small Grade 1 table, I wrote extensive field notes about their musical behaviours, took photographs, video, and had informal conversations with them. I collected any written reflections or drawings created by children that pertained to their musical lives. As the study progressed and a relationship of trust developed, I had an informal interview conversation with each child that was digitally recorded. These began during the fourth month. I felt it was extremely important to spend time with the children in their space, getting to know one another, prior to engaging in individual interviews with them. Overall, data sources for phase one included observation, field notes, photographs, video, informal conversations, student interviews, conversing with parents, ongoing communication with the teacher (e.g. conversation, emails, text messages), and *Community Arts Zone* team talk (e.g. meetings and research blog).

The second phase of the research began during the fifth month of the project. At this time, phase one continued while I began to investigate more specifically how children within the Grade 1 classroom experienced music in their out-of-school places. Based upon children's conversation with me in phase one, as well as attending to their musical behaviours throughout the day, I selected a small number of students to investigate their experiences outside of school so that I may develop broader understandings of them across contexts. I visited four girls and two boys in their homes to have conversations with them, alongside their families. This portion of the research aligned itself well with one of the overarching goals of the *Community Arts Zone* inquiry, looking more deeply at the role of the Arts within the community. In particular, my focus was to investigate the relationship between home and school and how out-of-school knowing of music impacts the classroom context. On a weekly basis, I became acquainted with several parents and interacted with them informally at the beginning or ending of the school day as they entered the classroom space. This provided a natural segue to visiting students and families in their home contexts. The families I worked with were very keen to converse with me about their family involvement in music, their understandings of how their child may use music in his/her daily life, and the overall function of music in the daily life of the family. All conversations were transcribed and member checked with the families of the children.

Throughout phases one and two, I also had extensive conversations with the classroom teacher. We had various forms of communication including informal conversation, emails, text messages, and video that she would share with me (captured on her iPad or iPhone) of happenings when I was not present in the classroom. At the conclusion of the project, I interviewed her in my home for approximately 90 minutes regarding her overall engagement in the *Community Arts Zone* project. She, too, had the opportunity to review the interview transcript.

Overall, through the process of drawing upon ethnographic and narrative inquiry tools, the weekly data collection generated a wealth of rich data over 6 months. I created over 100 pages of typed field notes, embedded with observations, questions, researcher thoughts, and images. These pages became the starting point for the analysis process. Filled with rich description and detail, these texts were critical to deepening my understanding of the inquiry. They provided information that I could highlight and reflect upon so as to identify apparent threads that were woven throughout the research process.

While phase two was an integral piece of the research inquiry, in the remainder of this article, I focus on phase one of the research as I begin to uncover the meaning within the many typed pages, providing a window into the Grade 1 classroom, investigating the musical culture. Through this process, two of the three research questions addressed are: How do children experience music in their daily lives? How do children use music to acquire French vocabulary? Pseudonyms are used throughout so as to protect the anonymity of the research participants. Interwoven with the findings is my own voice as the researcher – my thoughts, my wonderings, my puzzles. This provides insight into valuing researcher reflexivity, my reflections throughout that influence and shape the research process. These thoughts articulated throughout my field notes have provided a place and space to wrestle with ideas, both theoretical and methodological, as well as contemplate concepts about conducting research while making sense of what I observed and heard through conversations in and around the school context. Creswell (2012) points out that as ethnographers, being reflexive also means that conclusions are "often tentative or inconclusive, leading to new questions to answer" (p. 474). From Clandinin and Connelly's (2000) narrative inquiry perspective, they advocate that such ongoing reflection is necessary. They have termed this thoughtful attention as *wakefulness*. In the creation of my field notes during the ongoing research, it was my goal to honour both reflexivity and wakefulness. I begin by sharing some of my researcher thoughts as I first entered the classroom.

A window into grade 1

Wow ... here it is. The first day of data collection to officially kick off the music research project, exploring music in the lives of children as part of *Community Arts Zone* project. I am feeling a little nervous as I enter the classroom to begin this project. What should I wear today? How do I want the children to see me? Does that affect how I dress? What role do I play? Am I 'researcher', 'teacher', 'visitor', 'volunteer'? What term will the Grade 1s be most familiar with so that they may grasp what it is I am doing there? I decided that I would have the classroom teacher, introduce me as Madame Shelley. My mind is a flurry of activity as I am recollecting a lot of details today about the beginnings of my doctoral dissertation research where I engaged in a similar project in another province in 2006. It is so hard to believe that it is almost 8 years ago since I was involved in that experience. Time sure flies!

I recognize that I have some subjectivities going in to this project because I have the previous experience that I bring alongside me into this research context. I learned so much from that work with Grade 2/3 children. Will I have similar findings? Different findings? How will their in- and out-of-school experiences interplay? How will the role of the teacher affect this experience? How will the integration of French Immersion impact this experience? What about the literacy piece? I am excited to explore some similar, yet different concepts in another province, another classroom, another group of children, another grade, and the integration of another language ... French Immersion!

Some of the Grade 1 children may remember me from my visit back in the fall. I hope so! At that time, I visited their classroom to get a feel for the context, seeing if it might be the right fit for this project. It takes time to build trust with the children and I am conscious that I need to be present throughout the day so that I may engage with them in different settings and contexts. In order for them to be willing to talk with me, I need to observe them and participate in what they are doing in various spaces and places. (Field note excerpt, 10 January 2014)

Upon entering the Grade 1 classroom, I was greeted with vibrant visuals all around the room. From ceiling to floor, children's work was evident as it was displayed all around the room. Groupings of tables were surrounded by five or six chairs so that children could collaboratively work with one another. A large carpeted area in one corner of the classroom faced a beautiful, bright window. A large open space welcomed possibilities for movement, including classroom yoga. Anchor charts around the room were positioned so that children could reference French vocabulary such as the months of the year, days of the week, various math visuals, as well as the vocabulary words of the week. In several areas of the classroom, cubbies and totes provided spaces for children to organize their work. It became quickly apparent to me that children had freedom in their workspace. It was more common to see children working alongside one another on the floor or on the carpet as opposed to at their tables. On one of the blackboards, a list of children's names followed underneath five possible centre activities. The names, attached with magnets, were able to be manipulated and moved around as children flowed through the various centres throughout the week.

Three classroom computers were available for children to use, as well as 10 iPads. I soon came to see that the Grade 1 teacher, Madame Nicole, embraced and infused technology into her classroom teaching. She frequently used her laptop and iPhone as classroom resources, as well as projected lessons from her laptop onto a large screen. Children regularly used the iPads to document their work. By taking photos with the iPad and subsequently creating visual text, they often recorded themselves speaking about their learning. This was particularly useful as the children acquired greater fluency in the French language. Madame Nicole had a classroom blog she created to share children's work and inform parents about the exciting things happening in the Grade 1 classroom. She frequently posted photos and videos of the children. In addition, Madame Nicole set up a classroom blog for each child. Children regularly contributed to their blogs and had opportunities to respond to one another. It was fascinating to watch the fluency through which the Grade 1 children navigated the use of technology. All of these aspects assisted with their literacy skills and definitely contributed towards increased fluency in French as their second language. It was quickly obvious to me at how familiarized children were with the use of technology. I anticipated that my use of my cell phone to capture pictures or video might be a distraction; however, Madame Nicole reminded me that, "They were born with one of these in their hands!" While some children were occasionally interested to come over and see what I was downloading onto my laptop, the majority of time, children were not focused upon what I was capturing.

Music-making: infusing the arts

As the classroom teacher, Madame Nicole also was the Music teacher for her Grade 1 class. Having a Music teaching background, she infused a great deal of music-making into the routines of the Grade 1 classroom. Prior to being a classroom teacher, Madame Nicole was a Grade 1–8 Music teacher who embraced Carl Orff pedagogy and philosophy in her teaching. Carl Orff (1895–1982) was a German composer and pedagogue whose attention focused on the creation of musical ideas through improvization and imagination. Orff philosophy in classrooms focuses on fostering creativity through the use of music, movement, singing, listening, speech, and playing pitched (e.g. xylophones, metallophones, glockenspiels) and non-pitched percussion instruments (e.g. woods [woodblock, maracas], metals [triangle, bells], and skins [hand drum]). This was her second year as a Grade 1 teacher. Singing frequently occurred throughout the day while children practiced vocabulary and learned how to count in various ways. Occasionally, she would use a drum to maintain a steady beat to accompany rhythmic counting patterns as children developed math proficiency in counting in French. Madame Nicole also used singing and rhythmic chants during times of transition to move children from one activity to another. The children quickly caught on to these songs and chants and would frequently be heard singing along with her. I also noticed the frequency with which the children would naturally and spontaneously begin singing without the guidance of Madame Nicole. I noted that she encouraged the music-making and did not dissolve the musical behaviours that were evident in the classroom. It was not long into my classroom time that I saw that Madame Nicole's classroom space was infused with music-making across the curriculum. It appeared very naturalized and fluid.

Madame Nicole tied the children's musical understanding to their development of French vocabulary. She frequently would use the content of a subject area such as Social Studies or Science and develop proficiency with the vocabulary and writing by connecting it to musical knowledge, particularly by using the musical elements of beat and rhythm. By using one-syllable words (equal to a quarter note rhythm or the clapping syllable "ta") or two-syllable words (equal to the rhythm of two eighth notes or the clapping syllable "ti-ti"), children could practice both their language development and musical skills. An example of this was the creation of "La musique du printemps" where the children collaboratively developed a bank of vocabulary words about spring. The visual example shows a sample of a composition creation.

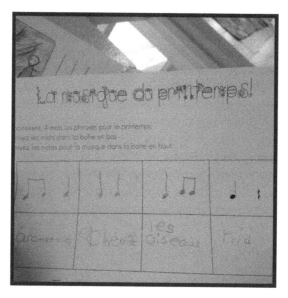

Figure 2. La musique du printemps.

Here, the children created their own eight-beat rhythmic patterns based upon the words chosen. This example demonstrates an eight-beat rhythmic pattern of "ti-ti ta, ta ta, ta ti-ti, ta rest". This coordinates with the French words about spring that were used: arc-en ciel (rainbow), che-nille (caterpillar), les ois-eaux (the birds), and nid (nest). The words did not have to be organized into sentences, rather the activity was about utilizing high-frequency words related to a theme. It seemed as though segmenting words in this way promoted the children's articulation of the syllables, solidified second language acquisition of French words, and also supported phonemic awareness. Children could perform these words through clapping or using body percussion.

Similar to this activity, while engaging in a particular unit exploring *community*, the class made a visit to a local ice cream store, which was within walking distance from the school. Following the visit, the children determined one- and two-syllable words that were related to the topic. Madame Nicole printed them out and these were categorized into various rhythmic

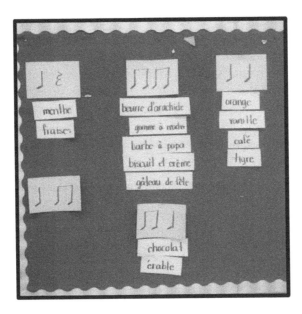

Figure 3. La crème glacée.

patterns on the bulletin board. Children could then use the vocabulary words to create their own eight-beat rhythmic pattern compositions.

For example, the word, "chocolat" would be rhythmically represented as "ti-ti ta" or "choc-o lat".

On different occasions, I would observe children working with their vocabulary words and attaching rhythmic patterning to them. On one particular morning, as the day began, I observed some children working together on the classroom floor, playing a game of *Memory*, where they were trying to find a pair of matching vocabulary cards. These high-frequency word flashcards were made by Madame Nicole. Without prompting, the children would recall the syllables of the words with the rhythmic flow with which they were familiar. In this instance, the rhythmic flow promoted accurate articulation of the French words.

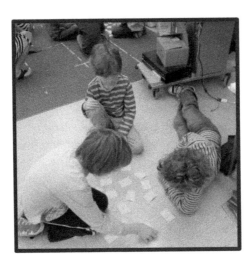

Figure 4. Vocabulary Memory.

All of these examples provided definitely tie to the research by Brandt et al. (2012) who acknowledge the entanglement between music and language that many researchers have sought to understand. They posit that language can be seen as a special type of music; in fact, children naturally attend to the musical features of spoken language.

As I began to notice these moments of how Madame Nicole infused music-making across the curriculum, shortly into my time in the classroom, I noted her response to my presence. I was fascinated that my mere *being there* in her classroom lent value to her role as an Arts educator, and more specifically, as a Music educator. After a few visits, I noted these thoughts in my field notes:

> At the end of the day, I asked Madame Nicole how she was feeling about me being present in the classroom. She said, 'I love it!' As she was tidying up the room, she paused what she was doing and looked at me and said something to the effect of, 'You know, it makes me feel *valued* and having you here makes me realize that *what I do is valued.*' I thought, 'Wow, it IS important!' She was referring to teaching through the Arts. We went on to discuss how I was feeling … that teacher preparation is so important and I recognize that in the short few days that I have been with her already. If you are competent in the content and instructional strategies, there are so many more possibilities for integrating the Arts across the curriculum! (Field note excerpt, 23 January 2014)

In addition to the music that happened in the regular classroom, Madame Nicole taught Music class to the children most often in a portable classroom outside the school. This room was equipped with a variety of Orff instruments. While attending to the provincial curriculum, her music classes involved engaging children in creativity through a variety of musical behaviours such as singing, moving, playing, reading, writing, listening, and composing. All classes were very interactive and engaging. By the end of the school year, it was astounding to see the proficiency through which the Grade 1 children embodied musical understanding.

Music on the periphery

Along with the many rich moments of music-making that I saw infused across the curriculum in the Grade 1 class, of particular interest were the moments that I seemed to *catch* happening in between classroom activities or during times of transition. These moments were frequently spontaneous and infused throughout the school day. These were mostly in English, yet it was not uncommon for me to hear children singing quietly in French as they went about their independent work. The majority of the time, the music-making involved two or more students. Due to the fact that the carpet area in the classroom was a common meeting space throughout the day, I often saw a duo of students engage in a quick handclapping game prior to Madame Nicole beginning her instruction. It was as if they tried to squeeze in music wherever they could.

Handclapping games were very popular, particularly among the girls, but also between the boys, as well as girls and boys. As springtime neared and the snow disappeared, these musical activities seemed to become more prevalent on the playground as well. Singing could be heard while children engaged in skipping games.

With both the handclapping games and the singing activities, what became apparent to me was the ease with which the students obtained accuracy in figuring out these rhythmic and melodic activities. The fluency with which these musical activities oozed out of their bodies was very obvious. Frequently, I could see and hear the children singing complex melodies that were permeated with challenging rhythmic behaviours, often with

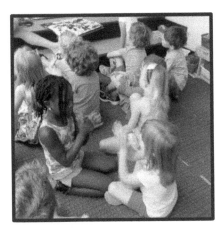

Figure 5. Handclapping.

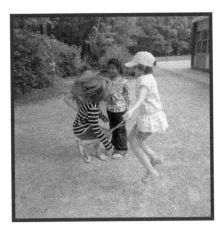

Figure 6. Playground Music.

syncopation and dotted rhythms. The children often co-constructed these as they taught them to one another. While I listened to these moments of music-making, I often found myself reflecting upon the school music curriculum, realizing that the melodic intervals and the rhythmic activities that the children articulated were far more advanced than what is outlined in the Grade 1 music curriculum. As the researcher, this made me wonder if this is unique to this particular classroom or if this might be the case in other classroom spaces. Thinking more generally about education, I wonder if educators spend more time in school teaching and reteaching children what they already know as opposed to challenging the knowledge and expertise that children demonstrate in their music-making behaviours, particularly children's musical knowledge that sits on the periphery of teacher-led instruction. This is definitely a matter that merits further thought.

Researcher thoughts: in the midst and looking forward

The frequency through which children engaged in music-making in and around the classroom context was very high. Music-making was valued by Madame Nicole and the daily involvement of music, both with and without the teacher, was more prevalent than what I had anticipated. What was most fascinating was the fluidity through which music occurred. It was always welcomed and it was woven into the fabric of the life of this Grade 1 classroom. The children were constantly singing their French vocabulary and using rhythmic patterns to remember high-frequency French words. In light of this, one of our goals within the *Community Arts Zone* inquiry was to focus upon potential ties between the Arts and literacy; connections between music-making and literacy development were certainly evident and confirmed in this classroom context. These findings align with others who have also identified the connections between music-making and literacy development (Brandt et al., 2012; Montgomery & Smith, 2014; Walton, 2014; Winters & Griffin, 2014).

Over the period of 6 months, there was a lot of growth in children's French vocabulary as the music repetition helped to solidify the French language. This finding is parallel to the scholarship of Zeromskaite (2014) who identified the importance of music's influence on second language acquisition; she described that music has the potential to assist in foreign language pronunciation receptive phonology and reading skills.

The conversations with the students led me to believe that music was so naturalized that many of the children could not necessarily articulate where the music started and when the music stopped. This notion is akin to Countryman and Gabriel's (2014) ethnomusicological research when they determined that children frequently slide along a continuum between speaking and singing in their multimodal vocal play. These ideas also resonate with Dewey's (1938) theoretical conceptions regarding the *principle of continuity*, making connections between past and future experiences. Dewey saw experience as a moving force, involving communication with others. It is my belief that Madame Nicole created a classroom environment that embodied and welcomed an ebb and flow of musical experience, both independently and collaboratively. Dewey urged educators to attend to the conditions of the environment that are conducive to learning so as to lead to growth. I reflected upon this ebb and flow of musical engagement in the following field note excerpt:

> One of the biggest realizations that I had from the conversations was this inability for students to identify when they moved in and out of music. It is so embodied, normalized, and fluid, that they often do not realize when they are doing it or when they are not. This was a surprise to me! I found myself thinking about how to help move them toward articulating their experiences. This is the first time for me doing this with Grade 1 children so there is potentially a challenge with them being able to explain their thinking as they may not have had the language to be able to explain it. (Field note excerpt, 24 April 2014)

Regardless of the children's ability to be able to identify or explain their musical engagement, there was a naturalized infusion of music which led me to believe that the musical culture of these children blossomed in this particular classroom space. The children definitely had agency in their musical learning as they often chose what type of musical activity they wished to share with their peers. I came to recognize that the children did not necessarily think in compartments of subject or content areas as they segued between visual, written, vocal, instrumental, movement, and speech work with ease. While this may not be the case in other classrooms, in this particular learning environment, Madame Nicole provided a unique and rich context for learning so that the children could move easily between these various modes of learning.

Drawing upon the theoretical underpinning of agency as a way to imagine possibilities for children to negotiate, create, and share culture with one another and adults, the children in this particular classroom were certainly welcomed to have agency in their learning. Ayton (2012) and Corsaro (2015) point out the necessity of children being valued for the contributions they make to understandings of the everyday world. It is my view that Madame Nicole valued the contributions that the children made for thinking in and across musical engagement. Thinking more broadly towards teacher education, this begs the question, How do we encourage children's agency with beginning teachers who are trying to learn how to teach musical concepts, musical theory, and musical engagement? While trying to balance pedagogical knowledge and instructional strategies specific to music education, how do teacher educators infuse a wakefulness (Clandinin & Connelly, 2000) toward a focus on the lived music curriculum – one that evolves based upon children's musical knowledge, skill, and desire? How might beginning teachers have an opportunity to live alongside teachers such as Madame Nicole and her students? How can experiences be built into teacher education programs so that beginning teachers see the possibilities that infused music-making may have for student engagement as they experience a rich place for music-making in their daily lives while acquiring a second language?

These awakenings and ponderings also confirmed for me, as the researcher, the importance of ethnographic research, in spending an extended period of time in a context to be able to develop understandings of the classroom space. By investing time in children and attempting to understand their narratives of musical experience, I acquired a deeper grasp of how to lay my own observations alongside the descriptions of their experiences. These notions capture the essence of living on the methodological borders of ethnography and narrative inquiry. With a foot in both methodological worlds, I lived on the edges because the classroom context provided the ethnographic perspective, whereas the more in-depth study of six children outside of school, offered a richness of studying the storied lives of children's musical experience. Both aspects were absolutely necessary in the music inquiry so that I could wrestle with tensions between my own observations and conversations I had with the children. As researchers, what we see and what we hear may not always be what children feel is most important for us to know. Thus, it is vital to study children over time, in the context of their everyday lives. These findings are in keeping with the ideas presented at the beginning of this article. In my doctoral dissertation study, I captured the essence of living on these methodological borders at the end of my dissertation (2007):

> It is important to remember that studying experience gets to the heart and soul of children's musical perspectives. Ethnographically-framed studies and narrative understandings encourage the study of children over time and they allow space for children's voices to shine through. I found that living simultaneously on the edges of ethnographic research and narrative inquiry allowed me to thoughtfully attend to music in the lives of children. Through such a multiple framework, I was able to look at both the school experiences of a group of children, while focusing on the lives of individual students beyond the context of school. Subsequently, over time, the children's stories told and taught me much. It has taken courage for me to stretch the boundaries between the ethnographic and narrative

lenses because such work has only recently taken its place at the research table in elementary music education. (Griffin, p. 191)

Whose periphery?

In looking forward towards teacher education, this research experience has confirmed that teacher candidates require time and space to be able to investigate their own prior experiences of musical understanding so as to understand how they shape future teaching practice. Vitally, they need to comprehend the importance of watching children over time to understand their narratives of musical experience. Opportunities need to be created within music education methodology courses for future teachers to see how music and all the Arts can be integrated to enrich learning contexts for children both within the classroom as well as beyond the boundaries of the classroom walls, extending to other spaces in and around the school context, home, and community. Teacher candidates need to be able to come alongside excellent teachers in the field, such as Madame Nicole, who can create and foster learning environments where children embody music-making.

Most importantly, attention needs to be drawn to those moments on the *periphery*, those in-between spaces where music-making is at its prime. I came to the realization that these moments that might be viewed on the periphery are actually integral to children's musical lives. It makes me wonder, whose periphery is it? As the researcher, the frequent moments that I viewed as being on the periphery, were perhaps, in fact, the core of children's musical culture, agency, and experience. It leads me to believe that my perception of periphery is not necessarily their periphery – rather, probably their centrality. While the music-making led by Madame Nicole was always vibrant, educative, and engaging, the musical cracks, the in-between moments on the borders of teacher-guided instruction, were spaces that definitely warranted watching and investigation. In thinking back to the underpinnings of children's musical culture, agency, and experience, perhaps the periphery *is* the space where these three theoretical constructs flourish. Indeed, as music educators, teacher educators, and researchers, we all need to take more time to notice the periphery and spend time in that shifting, liminal space of musical experience and possibility.

Disclosure statement

No potential conflict of interest was reported by the author.

Funding

This work was supported by the Social Sciences and Humanities Research Council of Canada [Grant number: 430-2013-1025].

References

Ayton, K. (2012). Differing pupil agency in the face of adult positioning. *Ethnography and Education, 7*(1), 127–141. doi:10.1080/17457823.2012.661592

Barrett, M. S., & Stauffer, S. L. (2009a). Narrative inquiry: From story to method. In M. S. Barrett & S. L. Stauffer (Eds.), *Narrative inquiry in music education: Troubling certainty* (pp. 7–17). Dordrecht, The Netherlands: Springer.

Barrett, M. S., & Stauffer, S. L. (Eds.). (2009b). *Narrative inquiry in music education: Troubling certainty*. Dordrecht, The Netherlands: Springer.

Barrett, M. S., & Stauffer, S. L. (Eds.). (2012a). *Narrative soundings: An anthology of narrative inquiry in music education*. Dordrecht, The Netherlands: Springer.

Barrett, M. S., & Stauffer, S. L. (2012b). Resonant work: Toward an ethic of narrative research. In M. S. Barrett & S. L. Stauffer (Eds.), *Narrative soundings: An anthology of narrative inquiry in music education* (pp. 1–17). Dordrecht, The Netherlands: Springer.

Brandt, A., Gebrian, M., & Slevc, L. R. (2012). Music and early language acquisition. *Frontiers in Psychology, 3*, 1–17. doi:10.3389/fpsyg.2012.00327

Campbell, P. S. (1998). *Songs in their heads: Music and its meaning in children's lives*. New York, NY: Oxford University Press.

Campbell, P. S. (2010). *Songs in their heads: Music and its meaning in children's lives* (2nd ed.). New York, NY: Oxford University Press.

Campbell, P. S., & Wiggins, T. (2013). Giving voice to children. In P. S. Campbell & T. Wiggins (Eds.), *The Oxford handbook of children's musical cultures* (pp. 1–24). Oxford: Oxford University Press.

Clandinin, D. J. (Ed.). (2007). *Handbook of narrative inquiry: Mapping a methodology*. Thousand Oaks, CA: Sage.

Clandinin, D. J., & Connelly, F. M. (2000). *Narrative inquiry: Experience and story in qualitative research*. San Francisco: Jossey-Bass.

Clandinin, D. J., & Rosiek, J. (2007). Mapping a landscape of narrative inquiry: Borderland spaces and tensions. In D. J. Clandinin (Ed.), *Handbook of narrative inquiry: Mapping a methodology* (pp. 35–75). Thousand Oaks, CA: Sage.

Corsaro, W. A. (2015). *The sociology of childhood* (4th ed.). Thousand Oaks, CA: Sage.

Countryman, J., & Gabriel, M. A. (2014). Recess as a site for language play. *Language and Literacy, 16*(3), 4–26. doi:10.20360/G2Q301

Craft, A., Cremin, T., Hay, P., & Clack, J. (2014). Creative primary schools: Developing and main-taining pedagogy for creativity. *Ethnography and Education, 9*(1), 16–34. doi:10.1080/17457823.2013.828474

Creswell, J. W. (2012). *Educational research: Planning, conducting, and evaluating quantitative and qualitative research* (4th ed.). Boston, MA: Pearson Education.

Dahlberg, G., Moss, P., & Pence, A. (1999). *Beyond quality in early childhood education and care: Postmodern perspectives*. London: Falmer Press.

Dewey, J. (1938). *Experience and education*. New York, NY: Macmillan.

Emerson, R. M., Fretz, R. I., & Shaw, L. L. (2011). *Writing ethnographic fieldnotes* (2nd ed.). Chicago, IL: The University of Chicago Press.

Griffin, S. M. (2002). *Music in the lives of children*. Unpublished master's capping paper Edmonton, Canada: University of Alberta.

Griffin, S. M. (2007). *The musical lives of children: A missing perspective in elementary school music*. Unpublished doctoral dissertation Edmonton, Canada: University of Alberta.

Griffin, S. M. (2009). Listening to children's music perspectives: In and out of school thoughts. *Research Studies in Music Education, 31*(2), 161–177. doi:10.1177/1321103X09344383

Griffin, S. M. (2010). Inquiring into children's music experiences: Groundings in literature. *Update: Applications of Research in Music Education, 28*(2), 42–49.

Griffin, S. M. (2011a). The social justice behind children's tales of in- and out-of-school music experiences. *Bulletin of the Council for Research in Music Education, 188*, 77–92.

Griffin, S. M. (2011b). Through the eyes of children: Telling insights into music experiences.*Visions of Research in Music Education, Vol 19* 1–26.

Griffin, S. M. (2011c). Tip-toeing past the fear: Becoming a music educator by attending to personal music experiences. In J. Kitchen, D. Ciuffetelli Parker, & D. Pushor (Eds.), *Narrative inquiries into curriculum-making in teacher education* (pp. 169–192). Bingley, UK: Emerald Books.

Griffin, S. M. (2014). Meeting musical experience in the eye: Resonant work by teacher candidates through body mapping. *Visions of Research in Music Education, 24*, 1–28.

Griffin, S. M., & = Beatty, R. J., Equal authorship. (2012). Hitting the trail running: Roadmaps and reflections on faculty informal mentorship experiences. In M. S. Barrett & S. L. Stauffer Eds., *Narrative soundings: An anthology of narrative inquiry in music education.* 251–273. Dordrecht, Netherlands: Springer ISBN 978-94-007-0698-9

Halverson, E., & Gibbons, D. (2009). "Key moments" as pedagogical windows into the video production process. *Journal of Computing in Teacher Education, 26*(2), 69–74.

Hammersley, M., & Atkinson, P. (2007). *Ethnography: Principles in practice* (3rd ed.). London: Routledge.

Honeyford, M. A. (2013). The simultaneity of experience: cultural identity, magical realism and the artefactual in digital storytelling. *Literacy, 47*(1), 17–25. doi:10.1111/j.1741-4369.2012.00675.x

Huf, C. (2013). Children's agency during transition to formal schooling. *Ethnography and Education, 8*(1), 61–76. doi:10.1080/17457823.2013.766434

Jeffrey, B., & Troman, G. (2004). Time for ethnography. *British Educational Research Journal, 30*(4), 535–548. doi:10.1080/0141192042000237220

Kinlock, V. (2007). Youth representations of community, art, and struggle in Harlem. *New Directions for Adult and Continuing Education, 116*(7), 37–49. doi:10.1002/ace.275

Kitchen, J., Ciuffetelli Parker, D., & Pushor, D. (2011). *Narrative inquiries into curriculum making in teacher education.* Bingley, UK: Emerald Books.

Montgomery, A. P., & Smith, K. M. (2014). Together in song: Building literacy relationships with song-based picture books. *Language and Literacy, 16*(3), 27–53. doi:10.20360/G23886

Van Maanen, J. (2011). *Tales of the field: On writing ethnography* (2nd ed.). Chicago: The University of Chicago Press.

Walton, P. D. (2014). Using singing and movement to teach pre-reading skills and word reading to kindergarten children: An exploratory study. *Language and Literacy, 16*(3), 54–77. doi:10.20360/G2K88J

Winters, K. L., & Griffin, S. M. (2014). Singing is a celebration of language: Using music to enhance young children's vocabularies. *Language and Literacy, 16*(3), 78–91. doi:10.20360/G2ZK5X

Zeromskaite, I. (2014). The potential role of music in second language learning: A review article. *Journal of European Psychology Students, 5*(3), 78–88. doi:10.5334/jeps.ci

Seven *chilis*: making visible the complexities in leveraging cultural repertories of practice in a designed teaching and learning environment

Daniela Kruel DiGiacomo and Kris D. Gutiérrez

ABSTRACT

Drawing upon four years of research within a social design experiment, we focus on how teacher learning can be supported in designed environments that are organized around robust views of learning, culture, and equity. We illustrate both the possibility and difficulty of helping teachers disrupt the default teaching scripts that privilege traditional forms of participation, support, and hierarchal relations, as well as disrupt static and reductive notions of culture. In doing so, we hope to make visible the complexities of leveraging cultural repertoires of practice within a designed learning environment in which novice teachers work to negotiate both common sense and normative conceptualizations of learning and culture.

Leveraging what is known about how people learn across everyday settings, we hope to contribute to scholarly conversations that center around how to create teacher-learning environments where equity remains both a design principle and an outcome of the adult–youth interactions in practice. We locate this work and our own orientation to it within longstanding research about the cognitive and sociopolitical consequences of participating in thoughtfully designed environments organized around expansive notions of culture and equity, learning and development, critical pedagogies, and design (Cole, 1996; Gutiérrez & Rogoff, 2003; Lave & Rogoff, 1984; Scribner & Cole, 1973; Vásquez, 2013). This substantive body of research has been foundational to the present work, making visible the possibilities for transformative learning in designed environments that draw on informal learning (Rogoff, Callahan, Gutiérrez, & Erickson, 2016) and "proleptic" (Cole, 1996) orientations to learning. Drawing on Cole, prolepsis' future orientation is central to design, as it involves organizing learning in the present for the future. Extending these perspectives, we promote a view of learning in which one's potential is not limited by her or his present developmental capabilities, or constrained by normative or commonsense views of teaching, learning, and culture that often imbue and organize educational spaces (Mendoza, 2014). Our design principles in this work support a future-oriented interactional dynamic in which the range of possibilities for movement and growth is undefined and open-ended. At the same time, we understand that the activity systems in which people traverse and participate are rife with contradictions that must be negotiated and made the objects of attention, analysis, and re-design.

Adopting this view of learning requires a careful look not solely at the learning practices of the youth or the teaching practices of the adults, but rather at their *relation* in moment-to-moment interactions over time. Drawing upon four years of research as part of a social design experiment, we focus on how teacher learning can be supported in designed environments that are organized around sociocultural views of learning and culture, and equity-oriented design principles (Gutiérrez & Jurow, 2016). In this article, we hope to illustrate both the possibility and difficulty of helping novice teachers disrupt the default teaching scripts that privilege traditional forms of participation, support, and hierarchal relations, as well as disrupt static and reductive notions of culture (Cazden, 2001). Specifically, we discuss how the default script and static notions of culture and cultural communities work together to preserve more traditional and less-than-equitable teaching practices that can serve to delimit learning and transformative forms of agency on the part of the youth.

Our experiences working with youth from nondominant communities as partners in design support us in documenting and addressing those subtle and often imperceptible contradictions that stem from the normative forces that shape and often reify asymmetrical participation structures in practice (Oakes, 1992). Substantive research documents the ways in which these racialized forces, driven largely by deficit understandings of low-income youth and youth of color, can serve to marginalize and delimit equitable learning opportunities for youth from nondominant communities (Ladson-Billings, 1994; Valdes, 1996; Valenzuela, 1999). Within this problem space is work that documents empirically how culturally relevant pedagogical strategies and practices can work to provide more equitable learning opportunities for low-income youth and youth of color (Duncan-Andrade, 2007 ; Ladson-Billings, 1995). The present study contributes to this important conversation by making visible the complexities of creating and maintaining an equity-oriented teacher-learning environment in which teachers organize learning activity in ways that reflect expansive notions of culture.

Learning theory in action: the designed environment of *El Pueblo Mágico*

The article grows out of our collaborative work with the Community Arts Zone project (CAZ) in which elementary age youth and pre-service, that is, novice teachers, play and learn together in an innovative afterschool setting, called *El Pueblo Mágico* (the magical community). In contrast to many educational spaces where youth and adults interact and the emphasis is on youth learning, the design of this particular ecology attends to both youth and adult learning, including new ways of working and learning together. Inspired by its Fifth Dimension antecedents, principally *Las Redes* (Gutiérrez, BaquedanoLópez, Alvarez, & Chiu, 1999) and protypical Fifth Dimensions (Cole, 1996; Vásquez, 2013), *El Pueblo Mágico* (hereafter EPM) and its university-school collaboration remain iterative and responsive to the ever-changing needs of the elementary age students and the pre-service teacher university students. Within this model, under-graduates (pre-service or novice teachers, most of whom are White) participate in a university course on cultural historical theories of learning and development, which are designed to encourage their attention toward practices of *learning*, rather than teaching – pushing against normative emphases within teacher education spaces. As part of their participation in the university course, the undergraduates join K-5 children, many of whom are from nondominant communities, in STEAM-oriented making, tinkering, and designing activities at EPM. Here the children have the opportunity to become the principal designers, rather than the consumers of the creative activities and games in which they engage.

Since the club's inception, youth have been invited to participate in a range of making/creating/designing activities, including but not limited to activities like *agent sheets*, digital storytelling, marble wall, squishy circuits, and garage band.[1] This playful learning environment aims to privilege hybrid language practices – that is, practices that value, make use of, and support the expansion of youths' complete linguistic toolkit – by foregrounding the benefits of multilingualism and heterogeneous and multi-voiced learning environments that support the creation of "third spaces." As Gutiérrez, Rhymes & Larson noted in 1995, third spaces are "places where the two scripts (that of the teacher and that of the student) intersect, creating the potential for authentic interaction to occur" (p. 445). More recently, Gutiérrez (2008) helps us to understand third spaces as collective zones of proximal development. Within this view, third spaces are interactionally constituted and traditional conceptions of learning are contested and replaced with forms of participation and practices that are contingent upon students' sociohistorical lives, locally and historically. Here, students' full linguistic toolkits and the conscious use of social and learning theory, play and the imaginary situation, are central to the ecology's design and potential (Gutiérrez, 2008).

As a social design experiment, EPM is organized around dynamic notions of culture, an equity-oriented approach to design and democratizing forms of inquiry in which mutual relations of exchange between youth, adults, communities, and researchers are advanced (Gutiérrez & Jurow, 2016). Of consequence to this project, social design experiments are guided by a more complex understanding of cultural practices creating the potential for more opportunities for consequential learning – that is, learning in which one's relationship to the material shifts as a result of transforming participation or engagement (see Beach, 1999). In this way, EPM, as well as the university course, is intended to serve as a learning environment that supports the development of third spaces in part by explicitly privileging expansive notions of culture and pushing against commonsense notions of what it means to be a teacher and a learner. To better understand the ways in which the environment is meeting these aims, we take an analytical focus in our research on the social organization of interactions within designed teaching and learning activity in the university course as well as in the after-school club. We do so in an attempt to understand better the challenges and affordances of leveraging students' repertoires of practice toward more engaging and consequential learning activity and forms of agency.

"Repertoires of practice" refers to the sociocultural tool kit that students develop as they move across time, space, and activity (Gutierrez & Rogoff, 2003). Taking this perspective of culture as it relates to novice teacher learning is fundamentally about understanding culture not as something inherent within a person or place, but rather as socialization within set of shared and divergent practices in which people participate and that impact the ways in which they make meaning about the world. Such a perspective on the relationship between culture and learning is also about attention to the "cultural mediation of thinking" (Moll, 1998) – that is, it is about organizing for learning activity in a way that recognizes the historically and socially mediated nature of tools and normative practices, and in turn their malleability and potential for reorganization toward more equitable ends.

Toward relational equity in educational practice: a focus on the social organization of interactions

Designing for equity, or creating the conditions for what we term "relational equity" in practice (see DiGiacomo & Gutiérrez, 2016), involves supporting forms of participation and relations such that the sense-making and repertoires of *all* participants are taken up and brought into joint activity in equally valued ways. It proceeds from the understanding that contemporary educational settings are organized in ways that privilege the experiences and knowledge of some while marginalizing, and often oppressing those of others (Moll, 1998). Contrary to often commonplace notions of "equal opportunity" within educational practice, racialized relations between a predominantly White teaching population and a largely Latinx and Black student population continue to shape and delimit learning opportunities for these youth (Matias & Zembylas, 2014; Nasir, 2012 2011). Working to design more equitable relations between adults and youth in diverse learning ecologies is the focus of our emphasis on relational equity, as we understand such relations as instrumental to creating the conditions for youth to take on increased responsibility, to shape the production of knowledge, and/or to contribute authentically to the telos of activity.

Accordingly, working toward relational equity requires more than simply attending to the unequal ways that racialized hierarchies structure social institutions and social interactions) – it also requires that those in positions of relational power continually reflect and reposition themselves in activity in ways that trouble the unequal status quo. To be sure, we recognize that achieving relational equity in educational practice is challenging, given the historically rooted and contemporaneously instantiated notions about the normative role of teacher (as expert) and student (as novice) – and amplified by the contemporary racial and ethnic composition of public school classrooms and programs. However, it is precisely within this problem space that we locate our ongoing study of learning and (in) equity in diverse educational settings.

To investigate the ways in which particular activities support and/or constrain relational equity in a designed learning environment, we directed our attention to the social organization of the interactions between the pre-service teachers (again, predominately White and middle class) participating in EPM and the youth (predominantly Latinx) with whom they interacted on a weekly basis. Specifically, we focused on the social relations in the organization of learning within a new making activity, to better understand how emergent forms of more symmetrical joint activity and participation, or relational equity, emerges in practice. In particular, this article illustrates our ongoing interest in designing new opportunities that recruit youth from nondominant communities, Latinx youth in particular, as core participants into new practices that involve more relationally equitable forms of participation.

Our emphasis on gaining better insight into *the relationship* between adults and youth as the unit of analysis in this work reflects our theoretical grounding as socio-cultural learning scientists – meaning that we understand the relationship itself as the vehicle through which learning happens (Vygotsky, 1978). We see learning as a social, relational, and culturally mediated phenomenon and as part of everyday social practice. From this perspective, everyday practices have transformative potential and serve an important role in helping to reorganize the relationship between cognitive structures and experience (Gutiérrez, 2016). Our work, then, challenges the dichotomy between everyday and scientific or school-based knowledge and practices and advances the important role that everyday practices, including youths' linguistic and cultural reper-toires, have in consequential forms of learning and youth agency development (Beach, 1999; DiGiacomo & Gutiérrez, 2016; Gutiérrez, 2008; Gutiérrez & Rogoff, 2003).

Examining notions of culture, teaching, and learning in El Pueblo Mágico

Fostering more symmetrical and equitable forms of participation involves shifting adults' notions of the youth with whom they worked, including their potential in the present and future action. Even in designed environments such as *El Pueblo Mágico* in which equity is an explicit goal, moving away from essentialist and static notions of cultural communities and their practices is difficult. Thus, developing dynamic and robust notions of culture is a key goal of EPM and its attendant university course, as how we conceive of people, their cultural practices, and our understanding of the regularity and variability in all cultural communities is important to the development of equitable learning opportunities.

By designing learning environments that introduce novice teachers to theories of learning and development and provide contexts for engagement in reflective practice, novice teachers can build a different pedagogical imagination – one that might trouble normative conceptions of what it means to teach and who can be a teacher. It involves and emphasizes teacher learning in practice. Explicit attention to reflective, mediated praxis (e.g. purposeful and reflective examination of one's practice through theory) is fundamental to supporting shifts in teachers' thinking and ways of being, as even more experienced teachers can struggle to find ways to recruit youths' repertoires of practice in activity. As human beings who live in predominantly segregated social spaces and institutions), moving away from essentialist notions of learning and culture is hard work that requires frequent participation in practices that are organized explicitly to push against reductive notions of culture. As will be discussed in our analysis of findings, in our own designed learning ecology, we found that the novice teachers' normative views of culture, in tandem with normative conceptualizations of learning (often instrumental, vis-à-vis teacher-led instruction), mediated the ways in which the activity was orga-nized – and subsequently constrained the potential for unbounded, less scripted, and more equitable learning opportunities for the youth. And as we illustrate in our analysis of teacher–student interactions, we noted instances of youth's culture being recruited in ways that did not support the creation of more equitable, transformative learning opportunities.

It is important to note here that as observant participants and researchers highly involved in the day-to-day organization and activities of EPM, as well as instructors for the teacher-education course itself, we understand ourselves to be contributors to the constitution of the social organization of the teaching and learning activities. As such, the subsequent critical analysis of the teaching and learning activity at EPM is as much a call to action *for our own* preparation of teachers to organize learning environments in more culturally expansive ways. To be clear, we see our own teaching practices as always in need of similar reflection and re-mediation. Re-mediation understood in contrast to conventional notions of remediation is more than word play; instead, re-mediation involves mediating anew and thus a transformation of the functional system rather than a fixation on individual people (Cole & Griffin, 1986). We should note here too that we take a developmental perspective on teachers' learning and view the processes of teaching and learning as being life wide and life deep and thus challenge straightforward, static, and linear notions of teacher learning trajectories (see Banks et al., 2007). Teaching and learning are iterative, recursive, and situated processes with ongoing and persistent moments of great challenge, alongside rich moments of insight, reflection, revision, and re-imagination. Working to change such processes takes time, support, and opportunities to repair one's own thinking and practices.

It is within such an understanding of these complex processes that we present our analysis of a routine yet illustrative teaching and learning event at EPM. Informed by a cultural historical activity theory approach, we see tensions and contradictions in activity systems and human interactions as areas for growth and learning. Accordingly, our analysis highlights moments, such as those when novice teachers fall back into the default teaching script, even as they are seeking to become different kinds of teachers (Gutiérrez & Jurow, 2016). And given what we know about the central role of human relations in the creation of collective third spaces, we aim to learn more about how to create the conditions for relational equity – relations that explicitly push against the multiple levels of asymmetry that inhere in normative adult–youth relationships in educational settings. Relationships, in the present day, that remain largely characterized by highly asymmetrical power dynamics along age, institutional, race, and class-based lines of difference. Again, because social relationships constitute and surround the *in-between spaces* through which learning occurs, we find it productive to attempt to unpack the social organization of the adult–youth interactions; with the explicit goal of unearthing commonplace and unmarked notions about perceptions of culture, which necessarily impact, and at times delimit, the potential for equitable learning.

Methods

As two of the co-designers of the *El Pueblo Mágico* research team for the past four years,[2] DiGiacomo and Gutiérrez have served as site supports, undergraduate course instructors, and/or participant observers for over five semesters. As such, there is a large corpus of data from fieldnotes, video recordings, youth and adult interviews and surveys that inform our approach to analysis of interactions in the club, which also includes the ethnographic data collected by the dozens of researchers (professors, post-doctorates, graduate students, undergraduate learning assistants, and undergraduate researchers) that have been involved in either a programmatic or research role with this multi-sited social design experiment. However, hereafter, we emphasize data from a singular activity on a typical day at EPM, because for this analysis, we aimed to uplift the sociality of discourse in action – cognizant of the ways in which broader social patterns are indexed in small discursive exchanges, as well as in the intricate relationship between perceptions of culture and practices of teaching and learning.

Serving as a pedagogical model for undergraduate pre-service teachers was a key activity for graduate site assistants like DiGiacomo, a role that required active participation in group activity. This form of engagement required a side-by-side approach to working with the undergraduates and the youth. In addition to this role, DiGiacomo also engaged in observant participation (Erickson, 1985), characterized by weekly descriptive fieldnotes and strategic audio recordings of interaction. For this analysis, we emphasize a sequence of transcribed discursive exchanges from an audio recording (with accompanying fieldnotes) taken by DiGiacomo on a typical afternoon at the Recipe Creation station during the Spring 2015 semester.

The Recipe Creation station – a hybrid science-literacy and maker activity – was designed by DiGiacomo to amplify the linguistic and cultural repertoires of practice that youth draw upon when engaging in joint learning activity with the undergraduates. The activity asked the youth and undergraduates to leverage their everyday kinds of knowledge about science, math, cooking, and language to come together to create, present, and test out their co-constructed recipes. This, then, drew upon principles of "making" (Vossoughi & Bevan, 2014), but also attempted to create a context of development for youth to develop new identities about themselves as learners and designers, as well as a context for novice teachers to work in new ways with youth, and to reflect on their beliefs about learning and culture, and about who could learn and how.

Approach to analysis

Investigating the social relations of a learning environment requires attention to the moment-by-moment interactions that constantly occur among the many participants of a given activity in a given moment of time. In the particular context of EPM, paying attention to the ways in which the undergraduate pre-service teachers discursively engage with the youth matters for understanding how they organize and mediate learning. Accordingly, we employed mediated discourse analysis as an analytical tool to make visible the complexity of people's actions, the cultural tools employed in those actions, including their social consequences (Jones & Norris, 2005, xi). The EPM social context was saturated with a multitude of cultural tools, linguistic repertoires, and a diversity of participants – in terms of age, language, experience with new media, grade level, experience with school, and ethnicity and race. Yet because it is situated in a school, we expect ongoing contradictions in its activity system, that is, consequential learning and mutual forms of exchange were (and still are) often in tension with features of traditional school, and their ideologies therein.

In our sense-making around how perceptions of culture interact with practices of teaching and learning, we aimed to employ an analytical tool that would allow for us to move toward a more nuanced understanding of how broader social issues are indexed by moment-to-moment discourse in action. Drawing on Wertsch's (1998) concept of "mediated action" as the appropriate unit of analysis, Jones and Norris (2005) argue that mediated discourse analysis seeks to make visible.

...how broad social concerns interact with the common moments of our everyday lives: to explain how discourse (with small d), along with other mediational means, reproduces and transforms *Discourses*; and how *Discourses* create, reproduce, and transform the actions that individual social actors (or groups) can take at any given moment (p. 10).

Mediated discourse analysis, then, underscores the irreducible tension between actor and mediational means (Wertsch, 1998). Similarly grounded in a sociocultural approach to the study of human action, we too proceed with the assumption that there is always a dialectical relationship between the actor and her mediational means, and more generally, between the individual and her/his society (Engeström, 2011). Studying a person's actions outside of the context in which it was given life can lead to narrow and partial understandings of human activity and potential.

Attempting to operationalize this perspective, we honed in on the discourse-in-action that helped to organize learning and interaction between Elena (a 4th grade Mexican-American student who describes herself accordingly) and her intergenerational group at the Recipe Creation station. Elena's group included her close friend, Alex (White 4th grader), three undergraduate pre-service teachers (two White and one Person of Color), and DiGiacomo, who grew up in a multilingual, Brazilian American family. Over the course of the semester, Elena's group had participated at the Recipe Creation station a number of times, but this analysis draws from a focal event that emerged on one day in the span of this group's participation in this activity station. We selected this particular event as it was emblematic of recurring activity at the club in general, as well as within this adults–youth ensemble.

The affordance of attending to this particular brief interaction led by Elena is that it allows us to unpack the ways in which word-in-actions are constituted by layers of meaning that must be accounted for in designing for consequential learning. Of import, these layers of meaning are imbued with and constructed across differential power relations. Because we are interested in the ways in which culture mediates the potential for the creation of rich and consequential collective zones of development – or third spaces – in educational settings, it was important to dive into an analysis of how particular and constraining notions of culture are instantiated through the social action of discourse in action, as well as how these understandings help to shape participation structures and, thus, opportunity to learn meaningfully.

How do you say that in Spanish? Analysis of discourse in action

In the diverse learning ecology of EPM, the notion of culture was taken up differently, by different participants, at different moments in time. This is not a trivial point, as how people make sense of culture and, thus, cultural communities orient them toward particular beliefs and actions that organize learning. In our broader work, we highlight the importance of understanding people's everyday practices, as they are indexed with sense-making processes, beliefs, values, and identity work. It is in this seemingly mundane work of everyday life that people live culturally and learn. With this understanding, it is not the purpose of this analysis to minimize or critique the contributions of the adults in the space – rather, it is to highlight the in-the-moment challenge in taking up and extending youth's culturally related contributions to learning activity in ways that lead their growth and development.

Consider the following representative interaction from our analysis in which we see how Elena began to create her own recipe by drawing on her everyday knowledge and cultural experiences. In this interaction, Elena moved fluidly between talking about her interests and hopes, making visible a variety of personally meaningful experiences which she appeared to relate to the current task of making a *chili* recipe.

Stanza 1

(Setting is an ensemble of undergraduates, elementary age youth, and DiGiacomo around a circular table with papers, markers, and cooking materials)

:05 to:45 s

Elena:	I like a boy in my class. His name is Ronnie Jose Gonzalez.
Undergrad 1:	There's actual butter here today, you got real butter.
DiGiacomo:	Yea, I did, we're going to melt it
Undergrad 2:	What are you guys going to make?
Alex:	Salsa.
Elena:	Yeah I'm going to make my chili.
Alex:	It's *salsa*. Do you guys know what the difference is between those?
Elena:	**Yea I do I'm *Mexican*.**
Alex:	Then speak Spanish to me.
Elena:	Oh *that* I can't do.
Elena:	*Chilis*, oh just kidding, 3… oh wait 7, I forgot 7, it's 7…7 *chilis*, 7 red *chilis*…

00:45–3:40

Recipe creating time, while youth are writing down recipes and drawing the pictures of their recipes

3:40–4:00

Elena:	**México, México, México!**
Alex:	Mexico.
Elena:	**Mexicó.**
Alex:	Avocados from Mexico.
Elena:	**Avocados from México!**

4:00–8:40

Youth are still creating recipes and adults occasionally ask them to translate the various components of their recipe into Spanish

8:40–9:15

Undergrad 1:	Ok so Elena your turn to share.
Elena:	**I'm going to have a Quinceañera?!…Ahhh….If I have good grades…**
DiGiacomo:	I want a Quinceañera.
Alex:	Too late.
Undergrad 2:	What's that?

DiGiacomo: It's like a 15th year birthday party, right... I went to a...
Alex: Do you know what your theme is going to be?
Elena: Uh-huhhhh [nodding yes]
Undergrad 1:   Okay so Elena you are still sharing.
Elena: Ok, 7 red *chilis*, 3 green *chilis*, 5 tapatillos, 3 tomatoes, 1 can...
Alex: Ohhhh, How do you say that in Spanish?
Elena: (mumbles no)
Undergrad 2:   Okay, how do you say green in Spanish?
Elena: verde
Undergrad 2:   How do you say three green chilis in Spanish?

Throughout Stanza 1, Elena openly said that she did not speak Spanish, and that she did not know how to say particular words or phrases in Spanish. When her peer Alex noted that she does not really speak Spanish, Elena did not contradict this.[3] However, these self-assertions about her linguistic repertoire accompanied her passionate talk about Mexico, including her proud self-identification as Mexican. She proclaimed her affiliation and knowledge of practices she identified with those of Mexican-heritage communities such as her reporting that she is going to have a *Quinceañera* (a typical coming-of-age-party for teenage girls) or her knowledge and her love for a traditional Mexican recipe, menudo. Elena's self-reported description of her limited knowledge of Spanish and her simultaneously held rich familiarity with valued community practices is not uncommon for Mexican-heritage youth, especially in light of hegemonic English-only practices in schools. Based on these self-assertions (in bold above), Elena, in her own words, identified as Mexican. And Elena lived her "Mexican identity" through her participation a varied and rich set of family practices that she animated in her talk.[4]

However, in this interaction, her identity as Mexican and her corresponding repertoires of practice are, for the most part, not taken up in ways that might have been more consequential for Elena's learning. Recall that third spaces are interactional, hybrid, and often uncomfortable spaces where the knowledge and expertise of the teacher-figure is not always privileged, and where the typical one-sided dialog of the teacher script is troubled. In the above interaction, when Elena talked about her *Quinceañera* and her appreciation of menudo while writing out her recipe, we understand her to be making sense of the task-at-hand in relation to her knowledge of these cultural practices. By expressing her connections to the practice out loud, Elena provided multiple opportunities for the undergraduates, and DiGiacomo, to take a deeper dive into understanding and potentially building upon her repertoires of practice. Yet rather than responding to Elena's declarations of self with curiosity and strategic questions about the *experiences* that led her to desire a *Quinceañera*, for example, or the settings where she had made chili or ate menudo, the undergraduates focused their questions on asking her to get through sharing her entire recipe, and on how to say various recipe words in Spanish. Such adult responses illustrate the need for teacher preparation programs to support teachers "development of expansive theories of culture, as well as to engage in pedagogical practices that extend students" thinking, engagement, and repertoires. These adult responses also highlight the challenge in moving away from more traditional initiate-respond-evaluate (Cazden & Beck, 2003) and co-creating third spaces even in a designed learning activity such as the Recipe Creation station.

The discursive exchange between the adults and Elena in Stanza 1 also reflects commonsense notions about what it means to be a teacher, in that the undergraduates likely understood their task in part in the interaction as getting the youth to share their recipe out loud. In this way, they were probably doing what they understood as appropriate, especially considering their social context–a school-based setting. Where the potential for meaningful learning falls short, in our analysis of interaction, is in its creation of a collective zone of proximal development, or third space, where the expertise of either the adult or the youth might have impacted the telos of activity or the co-construction of a new shared understanding. Said differently, while asking Elena to share her recipe allowed her voice to be heard in the group and honored her contributions, it did not extend or expand upon her sense-making. After she responded to the first adult initiated question, another one was asked and was subsequently answered without encouragement or the space to build upon the first response – a pattern of discussion that does not typically promote the type of back-and-forth movement that leads development. Of import, rather than unfolding in a way more reflective of its intended design (as an activity that could build upon everyday forms of knowledge and expertise), the interactional dynamic between adults and youth largely mirrored traditional forms of teacher–student participation (e.g. teacher asks the student to provide their answers, teacher moves on).

When Elena shared the design and components of her actual recipe (e.g. 7 red chilis, and 3 green chilis), the undergraduates transitioned into asking her how to say various parts of her recipe in Spanish. This type of adult response likely reflects their yet emergent understandings about how to leverage cultural knowledge, as well as perhaps what they perceived it meant to be a member of a particular cultural or ethnic group. So, they focused on their commonsense understanding of the language practices of members of cultural communities. However, in Elena's case, she had already made it clear that she did not speak Spanish, so asking her to translate at the word level was not a practice that guided her development or promoted an extension of her understanding. Nor did it encourage her to consider the historical practices and social relations that inform her present recipe design. At the same time, the undergraduates' responses may be reflective of the possibility that they were unsure of how else to engage her repertoires of practice other than to rely on a word-level translation request – again, suggesting the need for teacher education programs, including the one in which EPM undergraduates were a part, to focus on preparing teachers to engage culture in more expansive ways.

The larger point here, we should note, is about the difficulty in moving away from default teaching scripts, even in designed activity and within informal learning spaces that privilege mediated praxis. To be sure, the social organization of the Recipe Creation station did well in part to foster an environment in which Elena was able to take responsibility in crafting her own recipe, bring in her experiences, and express them to others. At the same time, we argue that we would do well to consider how to encourage discursive exchanges in designed teaching and learning activity that move beyond the traditional ask-and-answer teacher scripts, toward the design of activities that more closely resemble everyday practice. For example, in the case of the Recipe Creation station, toward the design of undergraduate–student interactions that might have more closely resembled the discursive patterns of a family making a recipe together for a special occasion – interactions, given the presence of more experienced adults and multiple forms of expertise, with the potential to reorganize the relationship between everyday practices and cognitive structures.

In Stanza 2, however, we see what we understand to be more authentic exchange between adult and youth, in which the adult expressed curiosity about one of Elena's experiences. This small instance of discourse-in-action reveals the possibility of opening up the possibilities of third spaces known to be critical to more consequential practices of teaching and learning. Consider the following interaction:

Stanza 2

DiGiacomo:	So what is your recipe? What are you making?
Elena:	Uh, uh, uh, oh, salsa. Sal-sa
DiGiacomo:	Where does salsa come from?
Elena:	Mexico, from Mexico.
DiGiacomo:	What do you think people eat salsa with there?
Elena:	Ooooohhhh, they eat it with their burritos, they eat it with their chips, they eat it with their menudo.
DiGiacomo:	hmm-mmmm, does everyone know what menudo is?
Elena:	Yea, I don't know what it is but I love it.
Undergrad:	**What's it like? What's in it?**
Elena:	It's sooo goooood.
Undergrad:	**What's in it?**
Elena:	I don't know, but I don't want to know.
DiGiacomo:	Why don't you want to know?
Elena:	Because then I won't be able to eat it.
DiGiacomo:	You mean cause you're worried about it being some…[giving strange face]…
Elena:	Yeaaaa [Elena smiling, acknowledging that menudo has inner animal parts…]

(Hereafter, action in ensemble moves into a different activity)

Elena contributed her own familial knowledge about menudo, bringing in parts of her personal experiences and linguistic repertoires. This interaction could have been taken up reductively with a focus on "oh all Latinos eat menudo or know about menudo"; *or* it could have been taken up in a way that acknowledges that she has a range of meaningful practices that she draws on to create her recipe. We see the undergraduate's questions of "What's it like?" and "What's in it?" as an instance of opening up a third space where the youth's contributions were more authentically taken up and attempted to be extended within the group ensemble. Elena found a way to make her experiences relevant to the making and learning practice, and while she was not able to fully explain what menudo is, she was not encouraged to move on quickly to responding to the next question. This discursive exchange more closely resembled an everyday dialog between friends – where genuine curiosity and interest pulled the conversation and all participants' contributions appeared equally valued because they were built upon. In this way, we see this interaction as moving more toward the creation of relational equity than we saw in Stanza 1.

To be clear, there could have been a range of yet more expansive adult responses and pedagogical moves even within this interaction. DiGiacomo or the undergraduate, for example, might have encouraged Elena to think about the practices in which menudo is a part, including menudo's elaborate preparation and the many family rituals therein. This richer form of engagement might have created an opening for her to bring together her own everyday knowledge of familial cooking with her emergent understanding of how to calculate the right proportions for a new recipe, for example. Unfortunately, given that the activity shifted directions at this point in the discussion, we are not able to know what might have been – but we lift up this example to demonstrate the complexity and potential in leveraging repertoires of practices toward the creation of meaningful third spaces in formative educational practice.

Discussion

Taking repertoires of practice approach requires a fundamental view of culture not as a fixed collection of traits or characteristics, but as a fluid constellation of experiences within a particular community or set of shared practices and histories (Moll, 1998). As articulated earlier, adopting and embodying this dynamic view of culture in practice is not easy for novice or even more experienced teachers who may be more familiar with understanding culture as immutable traits and in which learning is assigned a style by virtue of people's membership in cultural communities, (Gutierrez & Rogoff, 2003; Gutiérrez & Vossoughi, 2010; Moll, 1998). We reemphasize this important point because as Gutiérrez and Rogoff (2003) argue, culture is seen as inherent traits or abilities based on one's cultural community. Within this view, culture is viewed as homogenous and static and cultural practices practiced uniformly within a cultural community. In Elena's case, such a view would motivate one to assume that because she is a Brown-skinned young girl who identifies herself as Mexican, she must necessarily speak Spanish. However, as we previously alluded, Elena is a second generation Mexican-American who says she has little knowledge of Spanish. In asking her repeatedly to focus at the word level and to say various recipe words In Spanish, the undergraduates are focusing on more superficial understandings of Elena's cultural repertoire, instead of leveraging the knowledge and expertise gained in participation in valued everyday practices, including those imbued with her Mexican heritage.

As an informal learning space, EPM is designed to trouble traditional notions of what it means to teach and to learn. However even within such an informal learning context, we find that the pre-service teachers struggled at times to abandon didactic ways of organizing activity and learning grounded in previous experiences and preconceived notions about how adults are supposed to mentor youth (Kafai, Desai, Peppler, Chiu, & Moya, 2008). As a result, many adult–youth interactions defaulted to the same hierarchical power dynamics that characterize traditional classrooms. These power dynamics can be observed in the everyday interactions among youth and adults, among youth themselves, or even in the briefest of seemingly inconsequential discursive exchanges in activity. And because asymmetrical power relations have increased potential to reify bounded and less robust teacher–student scripts, we remain keenly attentive to their instantiations in designed teaching and learning environments. As we alluded to at the beginning of this article, working toward relational equity – again, relations in which all participants sense-making are taken up and engaged with in equally valued ways – is difficult in educational practice. But because we understand relational equity as central to the provision of equitable teaching and learning practices, especially in racially and ethnically diverse settings, we believe it to be an objective worthy of our continued investigation and designed research efforts.

Conclusion

Because our empirical setting, like so many other designed learning environments, is a social context saturated with a multitude of histories, cultural tools, linguistic repertoires, and diverse epistemological and ontological orientations, it seemed fruitful to employ the analytical approach of mediated discourse analysis that allowed for our analysis to move beyond the prose, and toward an understanding of how broader social issues are indexed by moment-to-moment discourse in action. Of course, as Ochs (1979) reminds us, transcription is theory and thus our rendering could be interpreted and understood in a variety of ways, and we would always seek further investigation and analysis, particularly ethnographically over time and space. We share this focal event and continue our analysis of such practices across hundreds of other interactions documented weekly at EPM. Our research will continue to pursue questions such as: How can we design pre-service teacher learner environments (such as this one) that promote openings for authentic discourse and different participation structures to create routine practices organized around relational equity? How can we support novice teachers' movement from more static views of culture towards more fluid and expansive notions of learning and of culture and cultural communities, including how to leverage young people's diverse repertoires of practice in joint learning activity?

Our work in general and this work in particular helped us better understand the difficulties in creating the conditions for the emergence of third spaces as collective shared practices between adults and youth in educational settings. In reflection, we offer a potential suggestion about how to design learning contexts that grow out of our longstanding, ongoing, collective work in Fifth Dimension settings – an idea informed by our commitment to the development of learning ecologies that privilege consequential and equitable teaching and learning. *Pre-service teachers, as well as more experienced teachers and educational researchers, should have ongoing opportunities to examine their own assumptions about culture and its intricate yet complex relationship with the social organization of joint learning activity in carefully mediated praxis.* We believe such opportunities hold potential not only to disrupt the default script, but also to rupture reductive notions of culture and what is cultural about learning that persist within even the best intentioned of designed learning environments.

Notes

1. Agent Sheets, designed by Alex Repenning (see Repenning & Sumner, 1995), was the centerpiece of an NSF collaborative study with PI Gutiérrez. The first iteration of making and tinkering activities were implemented with the help of Shirin Vossoughi and Meg Escudé (see Vossoughi, Escudé, Kong, & Hooper, 2013) and the Exploratorium Science Museum, San Francisco.

2. Gutiérrez served as Director, course instructor, and PI for EPM. DiGiacomo served a variety of roles as part of the EPM Project, including course instructor, and generated the fieldnotes that documented activity at the Recipe Creation station.
3. We do not know if Elena knows Spanish fluently or not, or if it is her preferred language; Elena was born in the United States, and we cannot assume that she uses Spanish regularly or has a strong command of the language.
4. We are careful to note here that these are Elena's expressions of her own identity and cultural practices; we are not advancing a notion of culture that is organized around food, fun, and festivals, in and out itself a more reductive notion of culture and multiculturalism (Gutierrez & Rogoff, 2003).

Acknowledgements

We would like to thank the MacArthur Foundation Connected Learning Research Network for their continued support with this research and the University of Colorado Outreach. We are also grateful to our Colorado partners and the youth and undergraduate participants that make up the *El Pueblo Mágico* teaching and learning team.

Disclosure statement

No potential conflict of interest was reported by the authors.

References

Banks, J., Au, K., Ball, A., Bell, P., Gordon, E., Gutiérrez, K., … Zhou, M. (2007). *Learning in and out of school in diverse environments: Life-Long, Life-Wide, Life-Deep*. Seattle: The LIFE Center (The Learning in Informal and Formal Environments Center), University of Washington, Stanford University, and SRI International.

Beach, K. (1999). Consequential transitions: A sociocultural expedition beyond transfer in education. *Review of Research in Education, 24*, 101–139.

Cazden, C. B., & Beck, S. W. (2003). Classroom discourse. Handbook of discourse processes, 165-197. Portsmouth, NH: Heinemann.

Cole, M. (1996). *Cultural psychology: A once and future discipline*. Cambridge: Harvard University Press.

Cole, M., & Griffin, P. (1986). A sociohistorical approach to remediation. In S. deCastell, A. Luke, & K. Egan (Eds.), *Literacy, society, and schooling* (pp. 110–131). Cambridge: Cambridge University Press.

DiGiacomo, D. K, & Gutiérrez, K. D. (2016). *Mind, Culture, And Activity, 23*(2), 141–153. doi: 10.1080/10749039.2015.1058398

Duncan-Andrade, J. (2007). Gangstas, wankstas, and ridas: defining, developing, and supporting effective teachers in urban schools. *Wankstas, And Ridas: Defining, Developing, And Supporting Effective Teachers In Urban Schools. International Journal Of Qualitative Studies In Education, 20*(6), 617-638. doi:10.1080/09518390701630767

Engestrom, Y. (2011). From design experiments to formative interventions. *Theory & Psychology, 21* (5), 598–628. doi:10.1177/0959354311419252

Erickson, F. (1985). *Qualitative methods in research on teaching*. Occasional (Paper No. 81).National Institute of Education, Washington D.C.

Gutiérrez, K. D. (2016). 2011 AERA Presidential Address: Designing resilient ecologies: social design experiments and a new social imagination. *Educational Researcher, 45*(3), 187–196. doi:10.3102/0013189X16645430

Gutiérrez, K. D., & Rogoff, B. (2003). Cultural ways of learning: Individual traits or repertoires of practice. *Educational Researcher, 32*(5), 19–25. doi:10.3102/0013189X032005019

Gutiérrez, K. D., Rymes, B., & Larson, J. (1995). Script, counterscript, and underlife in the classroom: James Brown versus Brown v. Board of Education. *Harvard Educational Review, 65*(3), 445–472. doi:10.17763/haer.65.3.r16146n25h4mh384

Gutiérrez, K. D., & Vossoughi, S. (2010). Lifting off the ground to return anew: Mediated praxis, transformative learning, and social design experiments. *Journal of Teacher Education, 61*(1–2), 100–117. doi:10.1177/0022487109347877

Gutiérrez, K. D. (2008). Developing a sociocritical literacy in the third space. reading research quarterly. *43*(2), 148-164. doi:10.1598/RRQ.43.2.3

Gutiérrez, K. D., BaquedanoLópez, P., Alvarez, H. H., & Chiu, M. M. (1999). Building a culture of collaboration through hybrid language practices. *Theory into Practice, 38*(2), 87–93. doi:10.1080/00405849909543837

Gutiérrez, K. D., Bien, A., Selland, M., Pierce, D. M., Nichols, S., Nixon, H., & Rowsell, J. (2011). Polylingual and polycultural learning ecologies: Mediating emergent academic literacies for dual language learners. *Journal of Early Childhood Literacy, 11*(2), 232–261. doi:10.1177/1468798411399273

Gutiérrez, K. D., & Jurow, S. (2016). Social design experiments: Toward equity by design. *Journal of the Learning Sciences, 25*, 565–598. doi:10.1080/10508406.2016.1204548

Jones, R. H., & Norris, S. (2005). *Discourse in action: Introducing mediated discourse analysis*. London: Routledge.

Kafai, Y. B., Desai, S., Peppler, K. A., Chiu, G. M., & Moya, J. (2008). Mentoring partnerships in a community technology centre: A constructionist approach for fostering equitable service learning. *Mentoring & Tutoring: Partnership in Learning, 16*(2), 191–205. doi:10.1080/13611260801916614

Ladson-Billings, G. (1994). *The dreamkeepers: Successful teachers of African American children*. San Francisco. CA: Jossey-Bass.

Ladson-Billings, G. (1995). Toward a theory of culturally relevant pedagogy. *American Educational Research Journal, 32*(3), 465–491. doi:10.3102/00028312032003465

Lave, J. (1996). Teaching, as learning, in practice. *Mind, Culture and Activity, 3*, 149–164. doi:10.1207/s15327884mca0303_2

Lave, J., & Rogoff, B. (1984). *Everyday cognition: Its development in social context*. Cambridge: Harvard University Press.

Matias, C. E., & Zembylas, M. (2014). 'When saying you care is not really caring': Emotions of disgust, whiteness ideology, and teacher education. *Critical Studies in Education, 55*(3), 319–337. doi:10.1080/17508487.2014.922489

Mendoza, E. (2014). *Disrupting common sense notions through transformative education. Understanding purposeful organization and movement toward mediated praxis* (Doctoral dissertation). Retrieved from ProQuest Dissertations and Theses Database. (UMI No. 3635879).

Moll, L. C. (1998). Turning to the world: Bilingual schooling, literacy, and the cultural mediation of thinking. *National Reading Conference Yearbook, 47*, 59–75.

Nasir, N. I. (2012). *Racialized identities: Race and achievement among African American youth*. Stanford University Press.

Oakes, J. (1992). Can tracking research inform practice? Technical, normative and political considerations. *Educational Researcher, 21*, 12–21. doi:10.3102/0013189X021004012

Ochs, E. (1979). Transcription as theory. In E. Ochs & B. Schieffelin (Eds.), *Developmental pragmatics* (pp. 43–72). New york, NY: Academic Press.

Repenning, A., & Sumner, T. (1995). Agentsheets: A medium for creating domain-oriented visual languages. *Computer, 28*(3), 17–25. doi:10.1109/2.366152

Rogoff, B. (1990). *Apprenticeship in thinking: Cognitive development in social context*. New York, NY: Oxford University Press.

Rogoff, B, Callanan, M, Gutiérrez, K.D, & Erickson, F. (2016). The organization of informal learning. *Review Of Research In Education, 40*, 356–401.

Scribner, S., & Cole, M. (1973). Cognitive consequence of formal and informal education. *Science, New Series, 182*(4114), 553–559. Published by the American Association for the Advancement of Science.

Valdes, G. (1996). *Con respeto*. New York, NY: Teachers College Press.

Valenzuela, A. (1999). *Subtractive schooling: U.S.-Mexican youth and the politics of caring*. New York, NY: SUNY Press.

Vásquez, O. A. (2013). *La clase mágica*. London: Routledge.

Vossoughi, S., & Bevan, B. (2014, November). Making and tinkering: A review of the literature. *National Research Council Committee on Out of School Time STEM*, 1–55.

Vossoughi, S., Escudé, M., Kong, F., & Hooper, P. (2013, October). *Tinkering, learning & equity in the after-school setting*. In annual FabLearn Conference. Palo Alto, CA: Stanford University.

Vygotsky, L. (1978). *Mind in society*. Cambridge: Harvard University Press.

Wertsch, J. V. (1998). *Mind as action*. Oxford: Oxford University Press.

In amongst the glitter and the squashed blueberries: crafting a collaborative lens for children's literacy pedagogy in a community setting

Abigail Hackett, Kate Pahl and Steve Pool

ABSTRACT

In this article, we bring together relational arts practice (Kester, 2004) with collaborative ethnography (Campbell and Lassiter, 2015) in order to propose art not as a way of teaching children literacy, but as a lens to enable researchers and practitioners to view children's literacies differently. Both relational arts practice and collaborative ethnography decentre researcher/artist expertise, providing an understanding that "knowing" is embodied, material and tacit (Ingold, 2013). This has led us to extend understandings of multimodal literacy to stress the embodied and situated nature of meaning making, viewed through a collaborative lens (Hackett, 2014a; Heydon and Rowsell, 2015; Kuby et al, 2015; Pahl and Pool, 2011). We illustrate this approach to researching literacy pedagogy by offering a series of "little" (Olsson, 2013) moments of place/body memory (Somerville, 2013), which emerged from our collaborative dialogic research at a series of den building events for families and their young children. Within our study, an arts practice lens offered a more situated, and entwined way of working that led to joint and blurred outcomes in relation to literacy pedagogy.

Introduction

In this article, we argue that relational arts practice (Kester, 2004) combined with collaborative ethnography (Campbell & Lassiter, 2015) can inform literacy pedagogy and research in distinctive ways. Both relational arts practice and collaborative ethnography situate the researcher within her field of practice rather than commenting from a position of difference. In particular, in our study, ways of "knowing" about young children's literacy practices that were embodied, material and tacit were brought to the fore through collaborative ethnography and relational arts practice. We were interested in small, sometimes apparently meaningless moments when children and adults were engaged in activity, drawing on Olsson (2013, p.231), who likewise focuses on the "littleness" of meaning making ... "the littleness that lies there and glimmers in its becoming underneath the large, noisy events" (Deleuze, 1994, p. 163 in Olsson, 2013 p.231). In this article, we extend understandings of multimodal literacy to stress the embodied and situated nature of meaning making, viewed through a collaborative lens (Hackett, 2014a; Heydon & Rowsell, 2015; Pahl & Pool, 2011).

The study involved a series of family events in which young children built large-scale cardboard dens, and took part in table-based craft activities. These events were researched collaboratively by university researchers (Abi and Kate), community research-ers (Jo and Tanya) and an artist (Steve). We focussed on what Kester (2011) calls moments of "learning and unlearning" (p.227) unfolding within our collaborative research. We collected fieldnotes and video data at each of the den building events. This data collection at the events themselves was nested within, and took place in dialogue with, longer-term ethnographic and collaborative research carried out in this community by the authors over a number of years. As part of the Community Arts Zone (CAZ), we looked at the intersections between participatory arts and meaning making (Rowsell, 2015) during the den building events.

Throughout our study, we focussed on what Kester (2011) calls moments of "learning and unlearning" (p. 227) unfolding within our collaborative research. This helped us to reframe what the children were doing. We were interested in ways in which the children's own ontologies helped us get closer to understandings of communicative practices, which can, in the process, challenge the idea of representational practice. Olsson (2013) describes how by coming closer to children's ontologies of literacy, representation fades out in the process, and "We might discover that children are challenging the image of thought as representation and reproduction through making use of sense as production of truth." (p. 231). This movement in and out of representa-tional practice was something we tracked in our own fieldnotes and observations. Kuby, Gutshall Rucker, and Kirchhofer (2015) concept of "literacy desiring" helped us to see this unfolding process more precisely as having implications for literacy pedagogy and practice. Our contribution to CAZ was to re-think the knowing that happens in literacy pedagogy and research with young children through a focus on materiality and colla-borative ways of knowing. Our aim is to present a lens that could help think through the relationship between artistic modes of knowing and children's understanding of literacy that was situated and drew on ontological ways of being and seeing the world (Olsson, 2013). In doing so, we de-centre the reader and the research inquiry in favour of a more situated and embodied understanding of what was going on.

The project team

Here, we signal what we brought to this project. Kate has a background in outreach work but became interested in children's meaning making through her work with young children in a nursery (Pahl, 1999). She developed a research focus on children's meaning making in homes and communities and has continued to write about this, considering the ways in which literacies are materialized in different ways across different sites (Pahl, 2014). Her work has begun to engage more strongly with the arts not just as a mode of delivery, but as a lens for understanding the world. In this she has been helped by her collaboration with Steve over time (Pool and Pahl, 2015).

Steve has a background in visual arts. Originally trained as a sculptor, he is interested in how children interact with space. This has led him to develop numerous projects where young peoples' ideas and concerns are centralized. He aims to foreground playfulness through messing about with stuff as valid ways to learn about the world and how to interact with it for people of all ages.

Abi has worked in this community for several years prior to CAZ, and has previously done collaborative research with Jo and Tanya, parents she met at the Children's Centre. Abi, Jo and Tanya were all mothers of young girls (five in total between them, now six). Abi has written about the experience of researching young children's experience along-side fellow parents, whilst also parenting her own young child, and the implications of this for relationship building, positionality and research lens (Hackett, 2016). Therefore, whilst Abi's research on young children's literacy draws on a framework encompassing multimodality (Kress, 1997), ethnographies of literacy (Heath, 1983) and the role of place in literacy (Somerville, 2015), her research lens combines these propositional ways of knowing with more situated, embodied ways of knowing young children from her everyday life.

Thus, as a team we recognized that we brought to our practice ways of knowing and understanding the world from the arts as well as from ethnography and a focus on multimodal meaning making (Campbell & Lassiter, 2015; Coessens, Crispin, & Douglas, 2010; Kress, 1997). As we communicated across the CAZ international projects through a shared closed blog, common ontologies across the projects seemed to include a commitment to thinking critically about the nature of collaborative research relation-ships with communities (Larson, Webster, & Hopper, 2011), an interest in the reflective lens participants brought to work across movement, music, photography and drama (Rowsell, 2015) and a taking seriously of the ruling passions of artists, teachers and students manifested through the arts (Griffin, 2015). In our project, we drew on arts practice and collaborative ethnography as methodologies for shared inquiry. We focused on emergent and uncertain moments in the data in order to think through understandings of literacy through lenses that might be unfamiliar or de-centring (Olsson, 2013).

A dialogic lens for literacy pedagogy

In this section, we outline ways that the arts have been used in literacy pedagogy. We bring in theory from relational arts practice and socially engaged art to show how, in our project, the arts was not a discrete entity (music, visual art, photography, theatre) but a way of knowing that informed our lens. In our project, the definition of "art" came from the practice of Steve who is interested in what happens when art does not focus on an object, but draws on dematerialized arts practice (that is, arts practice with no clear object). In this way, our understanding of art within the project defied a clear focus on 'the arts' as a separate entity. Steve brings a history of practice to the project, allowing the research to sit within the framework of 30 years of practice and exploration. Steve has drawn on ideas from socially engaged art to link his work to the everyday and to emerging social realities with a focus on "cultural is ordinary" and lived experience (Williams, 1958).

The field of socially engaged art, or participatory arts, has experienced a complexity of framing and range of understandings (Barrett & Bolt, 2007; Bishop, 2012; Coessens, Crispin, & Douglas, 2009; Kester, 2004, 2011; Nelson, 2012). One of the biggest turns in recent years in art practice has been a move away from the artist as a producer of work to the artist as a producer of conversations or relationships (Bourriard, 1998). Arts practices organized around conversations were the subject of Kester's (2004) "Conversation Pieces" in which he described how "dialogical" arts practices could be organized around exchange and collaboration. Kester made visible the way in which artists were working in ways that were not connected to material objects or any kind of output but were themselves process led and focused on reciprocity and exchange. This involves a "reciprocal openness," a willingness to accept the transformative effects of difference," (p. 173–4) within art practice. Relational art constituted a challenge, he argued, to views of the artist as autonomous within a context. Instead, Kester argued, artists were responding to "the nuances of space and visuality, of integration and isolation, which structure a given site" (p. 152).

The idea of "knowing from the inside" has been developed by Ingold (2013) in his work on making, to argue that there are different ways of knowing (see also Coessens, Crispin & Douglas, 2009). By bringing together modes of conceiving and knowing with modes of perceiving and doing, knowing is then something that is experienced bodily, materially and in experience and feeling (Johnson, 2010). Ideas from Dewey ((2005) [1934]) and Greene (2000) on art and the imaginative transformation of experience recognize the ways in which art can be a form of inquiry that rests on unknowing as much as knowing (Vasudevan, 2011). The value of the arts as a form of world making and a source of imaginative resonances has also been explored by Hull, Stornaiuolo, and Sahni (2010).

In terms of literacy pedagogies, creative approaches from artists have informed imaginative literacy work in schools where wider possibilities have been opened up through an attentive artists' approach. In the United Kingdom, this work was largely funded through Creative Partnerships, a large-scale initiative that brought artists into schools over a sustained length of time, with a focus on sustaining creative ways of learning across the school curriculum (e.g. Burnard et al., 2006; Heath & Wolf, 2004). Literacy pedagogies as developed within Creative Partnerships were informed by thinking about the way in which artists changed classrooms and made them more emergent, relational and enabled different kinds of things to happen (e.g. Galton, 2010; Safford & Barrs, 2005; Sefton-Green, 2007). Anna Craft and Bob Jeffery wrote about the concept of "possibility thinking" as a way of describing the unlocking of new ways of working that artists generated within schools (Craft, 2000, 2002; Jeffrey & Craft, 2004). Teachers and students were encouraged by artists to work in different ways; to not pay attention to time, to focus on process over product and to look differently at the world. Within Creative Partnerships, Kate and Steve collaboratively explored with children the impact of a group of artists in a school. Focussing on moments of "messing about" in the school day led to an understanding of how important in-between moments of creativity and improvisation were for the children (Pahl & Pool, 2011).

The encounter between Steve and Abi was therefore influenced by a genealogy of practice that included multimodality and visual methods together with collaborative ethnography (Abi) and a history of creative interventions in schools together with a situated and socially engaged art practice with a focus on making and play (Steve). The intersection of these genealogies created the space of practice that was CAZ. This relational quality has affinities with another key influence on this project, collaborative ethnography (Campbell & Lassiter, 2010). In that ethnography is a way of noticing and perceiving the world differently, through a particular lens of participant observation, fieldwork and interviews, collaborative ethnography, like relational arts practice, allows in a dialogic quality to the process of creating ideas with other people. This process becomes the methodology and the way of knowing. Campbell and Lassiter talk about processes of "reciprocal analysis," which open up when participants shape and construct the research space (Campbell & Lassiter, 2010). Academics can no longer "know" everything about a community, rather community co-researchers can frame and construct the field, aided by academics. Both socially engaged art and collaborative ethnography involve "unknowing" or a kind of radical openness to emergence and staying with a sense of what might happen (Vasudevan, 2011).

Perhaps the most liberating aspect of this theoretical framework is a de-centring of expertise; people "know" what they are doing and here the knowing is embedded in practice. Academic knowledge takes a back seat when encountering other more located or situated ways of knowing. To conclude this section, then, a literacy pedagogy that rests on "unknowing" and emergence involves something more than just the presence of an artist. The collaboration between the artist and the researchers, children and parents becomes a site for alternative meanings to emerge. This might mean a de-centring of what is known about literacy or authorities of knowing.

> One important attribute of works of art, and arts based research, can be their capacity for enhancing alternative meanings that adhere to social phenomena, thereby undercutting the authority of the master narrative. (Barone & Eisner, 2012, p. 124)

Literacy as embodied, material and within movement

Within our research, we were interested in how different modes offered particular affordances for meaning making (Kress, 1997). Work by Pahl (2008), Flewitt (2008), and more recently by Hackett (2014a) has encouraged a much broader notion of literacy that understands literacy practices to be enmeshed in other modes. Heydon and Rowsell (2015) argue that it is important to recognize "the reciprocity between literacy as embodied and literacy as grounded in relationships" (p. 469). They invite a perspective that recognizes everyday lived experiences and their sensory qualities as entangled within literacy. In her study of toddlers' literacy practices, Hvit (2015) stressed literacy as manifested in action, in things that children do. The educators in Hvit's study described literacy as connected to the children's bodies, through for example, drawing letters in a sand tray, and to materials, so that for example, holding a crayon indicated drawing, whilst the same action with a pencil was considered writing.

Ingold (2007), Pink (2009) and others have emphasized the role of movement with regards to how the body experiences the world through its emplacement. This framing, connecting body, place and movement, was taken up by Hackett (2014a) to show the role of children's movement in a museum in the production of shared, emplaced literacy practices. Our cardboard den events were dominated by the experience of place through movement. The children's creation of new spatial experiences took place through constructing and then going into the cardboard dens.

Significant to conceptualizations of literacy that rely on materiality and the body are new materialist theories that move beyond think /do and mind /body dualisms (Barad, 2007; Lenz Taguchi, 2010). Some of this work emphasizes the way in which language issues from the body, from tongues, mouths and vocal chords (Lercercle, 2002; MacLure, 2013, 2016). Connecting language back with the materiality of how it issues from the body would enable a reconceptualization of language as "a 'metaphysical surface' on which the very distinction between words and things is played out" (MacLure, 2013, p. 663). Somerville (2015) has stressed the entanglement between place and language, showing how the material world calls children to respond in certain ways, including through language or sounding.

Olsson (2013) has shown that children work with their own representational logics in order to make language. In the collaborative projects she describes, the children themselves experimented with ontological understandings of language.

> It seemed to us from our early observations that the children asked about the foundation of language as a representational system and that they enjoyed experimenting with that ontological question through producing new representations. (p. 241)

The located ways in which Olsson and her colleagues were able to make sense of the children's playful understandings of the world resonated with us as we tried to engage with the material and sensory engagement of the children with the play spaces. Kuby et al. (2015) have drawn on theories of new materialism to explore the role of non-human objects in literacy pedagogy in a classroom. They emphasize the role of time and space for children to explore possibilities of materials, such as how to attach pipe cleaners to a birdhouse model, in developing literacy learning. Kuby et al. are clear that such explorations with materials were not simple prompts or inspiration for later writing or story-telling. Rather the negotiations with the materiality of the pipe cleaners, the discovery that staplers worked better than tape to hold them up, was in itself a literacy practice. Kuby et al. (2015) conclude "we are beginning to consider the dichotomy of writing and intra-acting with materials as false" (p. 416).

This literature described above foregrounds materials, place and people's emergent inter and intra actions with them (Barad, 2007), as a starting point to understand literacy pedagogy. Much of this interest in materiality, affect and bodily sensation points towards non-representative aspects of literacy practices (MacLure, 2013). MacLure (2013) urges us to pay more attention to non-representative aspects of language and literacy practices, in order to re-attach words to bodies, to recognise the way in which representation "has rendered material realities inaccessible behind the linguistic or discourse systems that purportedly construct or 'represent' them" (p. 659).

In our study moments of a-signification or non-representation within children's meaning making seemed particularly resonant. Our approach connected with this literature on bodily and affective aspects of literacies through an emphasis on shared ways of knowing, between participants and researchers entangled in material and placed contexts. In the next part of the article, we will explain how these approaches and framings were manifested in a methodological approach. We then discuss some moments from our data set that seemed to offer a particular kind of affective intensity, a tacit sense of how we shared a sense of knowing the significance of what was unfolding, in ways that were embedded in our practice. In the following examples, we have specifically selected moments of "littleness that lies there" (Olsson, 2013, p. 231) that is, moments that resist powerful representational pulls or logics in order to further tease out how arts practice plus collaborative understandings can shape how literacy as a concept is ontologically constructed.

Context for the study

The purpose of our study was to connect literacy pedagogies with emplaced embodied experiences of families and young children in community settings. Working as a team, Abi was the university researcher who carried out the fieldwork, alongside Steve who worked with the children to create the cardboard dens. The other two researchers were Jo and Tanya, mothers from the local community who had done research with Abi before. As parents of young children, Abi, Jo and Tanya all brought their own children to some of the fieldwork. Kate provided reflective research discussions and brought her own perspective on the activities of the team.

Abi has been carrying out ethnographic fieldwork in this community since 2011. Her approach includes a long-term commitment to visiting and participating in this community, captured in fieldnotes and visual data. Since 2013, her ethnographic work with these families has become increasingly collaborative. In previous projects she worked with parents to collect and analyse field data together, through dialogic processes that emphasized the expertise parents have in their own children and lives (Hackett, 2016). Kate had also worked in this community since 2011, on lager scale projects looking at literacy in community contexts. Coming out of these detailed ethnographic projects was an understanding of language and literacy as materially situated and located in practice (Pahl, 2014). The fieldwork for this particular project centred on a series of four family events, each of which took place at a different community venue over the course of 8 months (summarized in Table 1). Each event included large scale cardboard den building, led by Steve, and other craft activities organized by community partners, including the local museum service and the Children's Centre. Each event was attended by local families with children aged up to five years old. At each event, video was collected using a hand held video recorder, and fieldnotes were written following the event. This data specific to the family events was viewed within the context of the wider ethnographic study, the long-term relationships and in depth knowledge of this site and these communities built up over a number of years. Table 1 summarizes, which members of the research team attended, collected the video and wrote the fieldnotes at each event. Our research team also met three times to analyse our data together, a process which we describe in more detail in the following.

Tracing the construction of the methods

When we got there, the Children's Centre staff were stressing that we couldn't make too much mess in the hall. Then they proceeded to get out tonnes of glitter for the craft table and blueberries for the snacks – the messiest combination of things you could think of! Steve, describing the third event during analytic discussions

Table 1. Summary of the community events and data collected.

Date and event	Place and attendees	Main activities	Data collected
November 2013 Toddler Takeover	Organized in partnership with museum service in the museum Widely advertised to all local families A group of families from the Children's Centre came to the event	Cardboard den building Soft play area Cookie decorating	Fieldnotes
March 2014 King Jack and the Dragon	Organized in partnership with museum service in a community venue. Widely advertised to all local families	Cardboard den building Craft table – making swords and crowns Rhyme time and book reading	Handheld video data Fieldnotes
May 2014 Princesses and Castles event	Children's Centre event in a school gym. All families who use the Children's Centre were invited to book a place for this free event	Cardboard den building Craft table – shields and crowns Dressing up clothes (princess dresses)	Fieldnotes Handheld video data
June 2014 Den building activity	Local playgroup session in a community centre Attended by the families who normally came to the play group	Cardboard den building Colouring sheets	Handheld video data Fieldnotes

Reflecting on their collaborative ethnographic research (Lassiter, Goodall, Campbell, & Johnson, 2004), Campbell and Lassiter (2015) discuss the potential for researchers to learn, be challenged and changed through collaborative ethnography. Pahl and Pool (2011) describe collaborative ethnographic work with young people in which alternate interpretations of the field forced the researchers to shift their lens, so that understandings of literacy were remade or re-imagined by the young people. We are interested in the possibilities of a collaborative, relational methodology to change the research lens itself; from this perspective, it is not only individual subjectivities which alter (Campbell & Lassiter, 2015, p. 6) but rather the way in which shared knowledge is framed and emerges.

Our interpretations of the children's experiences of cardboard dens were grounded in our own emplaced experiences at the den building events. During the events, traditional forms of data collection such as video making and participant observation were mediated through the chaos and business, our participation in running the activities, and, often, our supervision of our own children. As we looked through video data and fieldnotes we had collected at the events, these prompts evoked our memories of being there, rather than acting as evidence in their own right (Pink, 2009). When Steve talked about the blueberries and glitter in the above quote, it made us laugh, but it also resonated because for our collaborative research, our emplaced ways of knowing emerged from our time spent crawling on the floor, through the cardboard den doorways, in amongst the glitter and squashed blueberries.

In her book *"Water in a dry land"* Margaret Somerville (2013) describes how her own embodied experiences of her world meshed with those of her participants and with place. For Somerville, place-learning happened through her bodily engagement with the materiality of place; consuming rabbit stew, digging for grubs and massaging a friend's torn foot. These practice-based activities were the lens through which body/place memories were created, through which Somerville and her participants "thought through country". Describing "a methodology of lemons" (p. 59) Somerville explains how thinking about, handling and eating lemons became an everyday practice, a lens for thinking, so that "it is only then that I can know, through the lemons" (p. 60). Following Somerville, we seek in this article to outline an approach to collaborative ethnography in which knowing emerged from our emplacement and entanglement with the human and non-human world at den building events. This methodology of blueberries, glitter, cardboard and chaotic, embodied meaning making led to a reframing and emergence of shared knowledge.

Once we had soaked off the blueberry juice and brushed off the glitter, we met for a series of group analytic discussions. Vasudevan and DeJaynes (2013) propose the potential within the arts to making meaning in different modes, as a route to seeing differently, to reimaging and to "render visible the unseen" (p. 3). Taking a stance of unknowing and being open to "possibility," Vasudevan and DeJaynes ask "Who is being heard and silenced? For what purpose are we engaged in this work?" (p. 10). Taking up Vasudevan and DeJaynes' questions, and extending their proposition that arts is a route to seeing differently, we argue that our shared lens gave us alternate, emplaced ways of understanding the literacy pedagogies we observed during the den building events.

In the following, we present a series of incidents from the den building events. Drawing on the notion of place-learning (Somerville, 2013) and unknowing (Vasudevan, 2011), we resist drawing conclusions from these incidences. These incidents are not obvious moments that demonstrate "learning" or "engagement." Rather, we offer the "little-ness" (Olsson, 2013) of these moments, their inconclusive nature and resistance to categorization, as examples of what emerged as meaningful from our collective body/place memories as we tried to make sense together of what we had participated in.

Den building at the cusp of chaos

The scene begins with a shot of the castle and a path made of two narrow parallel sheets of cardboard which Steve has constructed, running from the castle across the room. Giggling, a little girl climbs into a wooden trolley (intended for wooden bricks), while her slightly older brother takes up position to push her in the trolley down the cardboard path. The trolley is too wide to fit down the path, so as the boy pushes his delighted sister faster and faster down the path, the paths falls apart, the cardboard becomes caught in the wheels, the whole structure collapses. At the end of the path, the trolley falls over, spilling the little girl onto the floor where she lies laughing. The boy drags the huge pieces of cardboard around the room balanced on his head, before running with a large piece of cardboard towards the open door out of the community centre.
Vignette taken from video footage, June 2014

When we planned the den building activities, we wanted opportunities that would be appealing to the children and child led. However in practice, the children were often reticent at the start of the den building. Steve was central to engaging the children with playing in the structure, by getting the older children to help with building the structure and then playing hide and seek with them. Often at the start of the events, the children were hesitant; they were shy to engage and did not seem to have many ideas about how to play with the den. They needed Steve in particular to mediate their engagement with the den, give them confidence and ideas for how to play with it.

At these times, we as a group of researchers felt a sense of disappointment or confusion at the hesitant and unsure way the children tended to engage with the cardboard den building, which we had conceptualized as being child orientated and offering open possibilities for creativity. In particular, Jo and Tanya noted the way in which the children seemed to copy each other, or do similar, repetitive things in the cardboard dens, such as run through them.

> Jo: "I'm usually keen on the children doing things in an unstructured way, but they only seemed able to interact when Steve finished building the castle and could engage and guide them."
>
> Tanya adds: "Every single child ran through the structure once, then went and did their own thing."

This sense of disappointment and unmet expectations resonates with Rautio's (2014) description of her reactions during a study in which she invited a group of children to do anything they wanted during a series of child-led research meetings.

> I expected the children to come up with all kinds of things to do in our meetings. I envisioned races with the toy cars, building things, exchanging things, throwing things, making up games and plays. Instead, the children began to imitate each other in a way that to me, at first, seemed like a disappointing and an uncreative way to respond to the situation; almost all begun to repeat and copy an activity that one of them had quite randomly initiated. (Rautio, 2014, p. 9)

Later, as their confidence grew, children's play in the den became wilder and increasingly bodily. We noticed that several times the play would reach what we termed "the cusp of chaos," at which point it seemed certain that someone would get hurt or something would get destroyed, like the incident with the trolley described above. Half a dozen children bouncing up and down inside the castle, banging the "roof" repeatedly until it seemed certain it would come flying off and the structure would collapse. Or a group of children dragging each other across the room in a cardboard "canoe" faster and faster each time, and releasing the canoe so it spins free-fall at the end of each go. Just when we were beginning to think we needed to step in and stop the action, things would simmer down, the children would disperse, leave the structure, perhaps wander over to sit at the drawing table for a bit.

Hackett (2014b) has written about a group of children imitating each other drawing on a row of padded benches in an art gallery. Drawing on Pagis (2010) notion of intersubjectivity produced through shared bodily interactions, Hackett argued that the children worked together in the art gallery to produce shared embodied experiences. Similarly, Rautio (2014) proposes the concept of imitating as a way of thinking about the children's similar activities as a collaborative way of exploring the possibilities of places or materials with their bodies. As the children in our study ran together through the cardboard den or spun together across the floor in the cardboard canoe, engagement with materials led to shared ways of framing and knowing the space. This diffuse view of literacy pedagogy resonates with Finnegan's (2002) view of communication as processes through which people "interconnect with each other" using "the resources of our bodies and our environment" (p. 3).

Den building alongside table-based craft activities

The main room for the event a bright and newly refurbished. On the right side of the room, Steve lays out his large sheets of cardboard, carefully balances his Stanley knife on a window ledge out of children's reach, and begins to construct a huge castle. On the left side of the room, a number of trestle tables have been laid out by the museums service for craft activities. Children can choose one of two craft activities, crowns or swords, and there are appropriate materials, some sample crowns and swords to show what the finished object should look like, and staff on hand to guide the children.
Description taken from fieldnotes, March 2014

At each of the events, the staff from the museums service and Children's Centre provided table-based craft activities to complement the den building. This contrast between the activities at the event gave us a chance to reflect on where structure and lack of structure sat within the arts-based literacy pedagogy of this project. Sakr, Connelly, and Wild (2016) outline the passionate debate between the merits of unstructured, process orientated art making in early years pedagogy, and what McLennan (2010) calls "cookie cutter craft," in which children are assisted to complete a predefined craft activity. Within this debate, open-ended arts materials and opportunities are described as offering children richer opportunities for creative engagement (McLennan, 2010). On the other side, it is argued that all art is a remix of what has gone before, and rich examples of children's modification of structured resources can be found (Lankshear & Knobel, 2006; Mavers, 2011; Sakr et al., 2016). Much of this debate rests on understandings of children's intentionality in relation to meaning making. From a sociocultural perspective, predetermined intentionality is used to justify the value of children's own creations through unstructured work with craft materials, as representing specific meanings and messages.

In contrast to this interest in intentionality, other research highlights emergence rather than predetermined intention in children's art making, arguing that the ongoing interplay between children and materials lies at the heart of children's art making (Kuby et al., 2015; MacRae, 2011; Thiel, 2015). In her description of a young boy making a rocket at the junk modelling table, MacRae (2011) draws on Foucault's notion of heterotopia to problematize the assumption that "a representational purpose" (p. 104) underlies unstructured art making. Rather, MacRae's analysis identifies that some junk models represented nothing, some began with a representational intention which dissolved during the making process, and some did not start with a representation in mind, but that some quality in the materials suggested a representation during the making process. Somerville (2015) notes the quick shifting in imaginative meaning making of young children playing under a tree, as dirt, twigs and fallen flowers become a cake, then a castle, then a building. As was often the case during cardboard den play, there is a moment-by-moment reaction to the materiality of the place, which seems at odds with notions of predetermined, fixed and invested intentional design. Kuby et al. (2015) debate how to term their observations of children's craft activities during a writing workshop. Rejecting the term "designing" because it implies an end product in mind from the start, they select the term "literacy desiring" to reflect the emergent nature of the art making, in which children "were not always intentional and/or sure about what they were creating in the moment" (p. 6).

In many of these examples of children's meaning making with arts materials, we note both the role of intra action with materials in moment-by-moment meaning making (Kuby et al., 2015; MacRae, 2011), and also the role of embodied sensations and notions of emplacement in how the children collaboratively created and shared meaning through their play with the materials.

> Standing enclosed within a column of cardboard taller than himself, peeping through small windows Steve had cut into the "tower," a young boy spun round and round, chanting "duhduhduhduhduh" stopping, and then continuing, whilst several children and adults stood just "outside" the cardboard tower, watching him.
> Description taken from fieldnotes, March 2014

In this case, the child could be understood as intra acting with the cardboard, yet the wider context of children, adults, place and materials also all played a role in the emplaced ways of knowing and experiencing cardboard dens, which were collaboratively produced during this episode.

Reflection

We have resisted a neat analysis of the children's activities but instead, opened up more questions about how we "know" in relation to literacy pedagogy using an arts research lens. Drawing on Somerville's (2013) notion of place-learning as central to generation of collective ways of knowing between researchers and participants, we propose that our methodology was one of blueberries and glitter, playing out on the floor of the Children's Centre and inside the cardboard dens themselves. Knowing within our research emerged from our emplacement and entanglement with the people and materials at the family events. The children and adults (including the research team) knew through their emergent meaning making with the cardboard and craft materials, as new possibilities for intra-acting with the materials came into focus each moment through the children's playing and experiencing.

Kester (2004) traces the possibilities of relational arts practice to enable people to collaboratively look in new, more open and perhaps more critical ways at their worlds. What emerged dialogically through our collaborative lens as our project progressed was a growing sense that there were ways of being with children which are authorized and validated by policy, and then there are these other ways of being with children, which feel more dimensional, real, that resonate with how we actually are, but that are hidden, whispered voices. These ways of knowing resist neat explanation, rationality or academic authority.

In Kuby et al.'s paper (Kuby et al., 2015), Tara the teacher describes her unease as the giant giraffe sculpture that her class has made is about to "go public" by being displayed in the school hall. Feeling a sense of needing to justify her teaching practice, she had told colleagues that her classes' exploration with craft materials happened "'in between' the required expectations, perhaps as a way to justify my actions" (p. 413). We are interested in Tara's sense of unease (Kuby et al., 2015), in Rautio's (2014) sense of confusion and disappointment at what the children chose to do, and in Vasudevan and DeJaynes (2013) proposition that arts are a route to re-imagining. Within our own study, the moments of children playing in the cardboard den, ploughing down the structure with the bricks trolley and sitting at tables making glittery crowns that emerged dialogically through our collaborative analysis seem significant in their "littleness" (Olsson, 2013), in their refusal to fit and provide convincing examples of the power of the arts as a panacea to teaching and learning literacy.

Conclusion

The "littleness" (Olsson, 2013, p. 231) of these moments led us to reframe our lens for understanding what literacy is (Pahl & Pool, 2011). This lens, drawing on notions of unknowing (Vasudevan, 2011) encompassed the parent's, children's and research team's ways of knowing and making, the histories of the practices of the researchers and artist and the cardboard, oil pastels, glitter and embodied sensations of being in place with, which we all interacted. It was through this framework that we observed emplaced literacy practices emerging.

In this article we have discussed how ethnography and arts practice worked together. We feel that the CAZ allowed the coming together both of individuals and disciplines. This project allowed us to work together in a way in which no disciplinary perspective took priority and each participant's ways of knowing were given voice in specific and relational contexts. Ingold (2014) describes anthropology as being about the potential to "do with" and a practice that is concerned with intentionally living with others. Somerville (2013) describes research as a meshing of her body and world with her participants and with place. We attempted to work in this way, and we think this way of working has potential to open up new emergent spaces where interesting things can happen.

Our framework for literacy pedagogy encompassed our adult and child collaborators and their and our engagement with materials and place. It allowed us to understand the ways in which children themselves can contribute to ontological understandings of literacy and language through engagement with materials and within and between our own under-standings and realizations (Olsson, 2013). These insights were connected to a pedagogy of unknowing (Vasudevan, 2011), the agency of materials within processes (Lenz Taguchi, 2010; Rautio, 2014) and an understanding that the processes of making were themselves forms of thought (Ingold, 2013). This then pushes the field of literacy and language away from strongly representational forms and towards knowing from the inside, and acknowl-edging the ways in which we might come to know through place, body and materials.

Acknowledgements

We are indebted to Tanya Evans and Jo Magagula, community researchers who were an integral part of the team. Thank you to the museum and Children's Centre staff, and all the families who came and played cardboard dens with us.

Disclosure statement

No potential conflict of interest was reported by the authors.

Funding

This work was supported by ESRC [grant number ES/K002686/1] and the Social Sciences and Humanities Research Council of Canada [grant number 430-2013-1025].

References

Barad, K. (2007). *Meeting the universe halfway*. Durham, NC: Duke Press.

Barrett, E., & Bolt, B. (2007). *Practice as research*. Chippenham: UK I.B. Tauris and Co.

Barone, T., & Eisner, E. (2012). *Arts based research*. London: Sage.

Bourriard, N. (1998). *Relational aesthetics*. Paris: Les Presse Du Reel.

Bishop, C. (2012). *Artificial hells: Participatory art and the politics of spectatorship*. London: Verso.

Burnard, P., Craft, A., Cremin, T., Duffy, B., Hanson, R., & Keene, R. (2006). Documenting possibility thinking: A journey of collaborative inquiry. *International Journal of Early Years Education, 14*(3), 243–262. doi:10.1080/09669760600880001

Campbell, E., & Lassiter, L. E. (2010). From collaborative ethnography to collaborative pedagogy: Reflections on the other side of middletown project and community-university research partnerships. *Anthropology and Education Quarterly, 41*(4), 370–385. doi:10.1111/j.1548-1492.2010.01098.x

Campbell, E., & Lassiter, L. E. (2015). *Doing ethnography today: Theories, methods, exercises*. West Sussex: Wiley-Blackwell.

Coessens, K., Crispin, D., & Douglas, A. (2009). *The artistic turn: A manifesto*. Ghent: The Orpheus Institute.

Craft, A. (2000). *Creativity across the primary curriculum: Framing and developing practice*. London: Routledge.

Craft, A. (2002). *Creativity and early years education*. London: Continuum.

Dewey, J. ((2005) [1934]). *Art as experience*. New York: Perigee.

Finnegan, R. (2002). *Communicating. The multiple modes of human interconnection*. London: Routledge.

Flewitt, R. (2008). Multimodal literacies. In J. Marsh & E. Hallet (Eds.), *Desirable literacies: Approaches to language and literacy in the early years* (pp. 140–161). London: Sage.

Galton, M. (2010). Going with the flow or back to normal? The impact of creative practitioners in schools and classrooms. *Research Papers in Education, 25*, 355–375. 10.1080/02671520903082429

Greene, M. (2000). *Releasing the imagination: Essays on education, the arts and social change*. San Francisco, CA: Jossey-Bass.

Griffin, S. M. (2015) Tip-toeing past the fear: Becoming a music educator by attending to personal music experiences. *Narrative Inquiries into Curriculum Making in Teacher Education*, 169–192. doi:10.1108/S1479-3687(2011)00000130012

Hackett, A. (2014a). Zigging and zooming all over the place: Young children's meaning making and movement in the museum. *Journal of Early Childhood Literacy*, *14*(1), 5–27. doi:10.1177/1468798412453730

Hackett, A. (2014b). *How do families with young children (2-4 years old) make meaning in a museum?* Unpublished thesis.

Hackett, A. (2016). Parents as researchers. Collaborative ethnography with parents. *Qualitative research*. doi:10.1177/1468794116672913

Heath, S. B. (1983). *Ways with words: Language, life, and work in communities and classrooms.* Cambridge: Cambridge University Press.

Heath, S. B., & Wolf, S. (2004). *Visual learning in the community school.* London: Creative Partnerships.

Heydon, R., & Rowsell, J. (2015). Phenomenology and literacy studies. In J. Rowsell & K. Pahl (Eds.), *The routledge handbook of literacy studies* (pp. 454–472). London: Routledge.

Hull, G., Stornaiuolo, A., & Sahni, U. (2010). Cultural citizenship and cosmopolitan practice: Global youth communicate online. *English Education*, *42*(4), 331–367.

Hvit, S. (2015). Literacy events in toddler groups: Preschool educators' talk about their work with literacy among toddlers. *Journal of Early Childhood Literacy*, *15*(3), 311–330. doi:10.1177/1468798414526427

Ingold, T. (2007). *Lines. A brief history.* London: Routledge.

Ingold, T. (2013). *Making: Anthropology, archaeology, art and architecture.* London: Routledge.

Ingold, T. (2014). That's enough about ethnography. *Hau: Journal of Ethnographic Theory*, *4*(1), 383–395. doi:10.14318/hau4.1.021

Jeffrey, B., & Craft, A. (2004). Creative teaching and teaching for creativity: Distinctions and relationships. *Educational Studies*, *30*(1), 77–87. doi:10.1080/0305569032000159750

Johnson, M. (2010). Embodied knowing through art. In M. Biggs & H. Karlsson (Eds.), *The Routledge Companion to Research in the Arts* (pp. 141–152). London: Routledge.

Kester, G. (2004). *Conversation pieces: Community and communication in modern art.* Berkeley: University of California Press.

Kester, G. (2011). *The one and the many: Contemporary collaborative art in a global context.* Durham: Duke University Press.

Kress, G. (1997). *Before writing. Rethinking paths to literacy.* London: Routledge.

Kuby, C. R., Gutshall Rucker, T., & Kirchhofer, J. M. (2015). 'Go be a writer!': Intra-activity with materials, time and space in literacy learning. *Journal of Early Childhood Literacy*, *15*(3), 394–419. doi:10.1177/1468798414566702

Lassiter, L. E., Goodall, H., Campbell, E., & Johnson, M. N. (2004). *The other side of middletown: Exploring Muncie's African American community.* Walnut Creek, CA: AltaMira Press.

Lankshear, C., & Knobel, M. (2006). *New literacies: Everyday practices and classroom learning.* Maidenhead: Open University Press.

Larson, J., Webster, S., & Hopper, M. (2011). Community coauthoring: Whose voice remains? *Anthropology and Education Quarterly*, *42*(2), 134–153. doi:10.1111/j.1548-1492.2011.01121.x

Lenz Taguchi, H. (2010). *Going Beyond the theory/practice divide in early childhood education. Introducing an intra active pedagogy.* Oxon: Routledge.

Lercercle, J. (2002). *Deleuze and language.* Palgrave Macmillan: Basingstoke.

MacLure, M. (2013). Researching without representation? Language and materiality in post-qualitative methodology. *International Journal of Qualitative Studies in Education*, *26*(6), 658–667. doi:10.1080/09518398.2013.788755

MacLure, M. (2016). The refrain of the A-Grammatical child: Finding another language in/for qualitative research. *Cultural Studies - Critical Methodologies*. 16(2), 173-182.

MacRae, C. (2011). Making Payton's rocket: Heterotopia and lines of flight. *International Journal of Art & Design Education*, *30*(1), 102–112. doi:10.1111/j.1476-8070.2011.01686.x

Mavers, D. (2011). *Children's drawing and writing: The remarkable in the unremarkable*. London: Routledge.

McLennan, D. M. P. (2010). Process or product? The argument for aesthetic exploration in the early years. *Early Childhood Education Journal, 38*(2), 81–85. doi:10.1007/s10643-010-0411-3

Nelson, R. (2012). *Practice as research in the arts*. Basingstoke: Palgrave MacMillan.

Olsson, L. H. (2013). Taking children's questions seriously: The need for creative thought. *Global Studies of Childhood, 3*(3), 230–253. doi:10.2304/gsch.2013.3.3.230

Pagis, M. (2010). Producing intersubjectivity in silence: An ethnographic study of meditation practice. *Ethnography, 11*(2), 309–328. doi:10.1177/1466138109339041

Pahl, K. (1999). *Transformations: Children´s meaning making in a nursery*. Stoke on Trent: Trentham Books.

Pahl, K. (2008). Looking with a different eye: Creativity and literacy in the early years. In J. Marsh & E. Hallet (Eds.), *Desirable literacies: Approaches to language and literacy in the early years* (pp. 140–161). London: Sage.

Pahl, K., & Pool, S. (2011). 'Living your life because it's the only life you've got': Participatory research as a site for discovery in a creative project in a primary school in Thurnscoe UK. *Qualitative Research Journal, 11*(2), 17–37. doi:10.3316/QRJ1102017

Pahl, K. (2014). *Materializing literacies in communities: The uses of literacy revisited*. London: Bloomsbury.

Pink, S. (2009). *Doing sensory ethnography*. London: Sage.

Pool, S., & Pahl, K. (2015). The work of art in the age of mechanical co-production. In D. O'Brien & P. Mathews (Eds.), *After urban regeneration: Communities policy and place* (pp. 79–94). Bristol: Policy Press.

Rautio, P. (2014). Mingling and imitating in producing spaces for knowing and being: Insights from a finnish study of child–matter intra-action. *Childhood, 21*(4), 461–474. doi:10.1177/0907568213496653

Rowsell, J. (2015). Same meaning, different production. In E. Stirling & D. Yamada-Rice (Eds.), *Visual methods with children and young people* (pp. 17–28). London: Palgrave Macmillan.

Safford, K., & Barrs, M. (2005). *Creativity and literacy-many routes to meaning: Children's language and literacy learning in creative arts projects*. London: CLPE.

Sakr, M., Connelly, V., & Wild, M. (2016). Imitative or Iconoclastic? How young children use ready-made images in digital art. *International Journal of Art and Design Education*. doi:10.1111/jade.12104/full

Sefton-Green, J. (2007). Evaluating creative partnerships: The challenge of defining impact. In *This much we know Thinkpiece: The challenge of defining impact*. London: Creative Partnerships, Arts Council England.

Somerville, M. (2013). *Water in a dry land: Place-learning through art and story*. London: Routledge.

Somerville, M. (2015). Emergent literacies in 'the land of do anything you want'. In M. Somerville & M. Green (Eds.), *Children, place and sustainability* (pp. 106–125). New York: Palgrave Macmillan.

Thiel, J. (2015). Vibrant matter: The intra-active role of objects in the construction of young children's literacies. *Literacy Research: Theory, Method and Practice, 64*, 112–131.

Vasudevan, L. (2011). An invitation to unknowing. *Teachers College Record, 113*(6), 1154–1174.

Vasudevan, L., & DeJaynes, T. (2013). Becoming "Not Yet". Adolescents making and remaking themselves in art-full spaces. In L. Vasudevan & T. DeJaynes (Eds.), *Arts, media and justice: Multimodal explorations with youth* (pp. 10–26). New York: Peter Lang.

Williams, R. (1958). *Culture and society* (pp. 1780–1950). London: Chatto and Windus.

Moving parts in imagined spaces: community arts zone's movement project

Jennifer Rowsell and Glenys McQueen-Fuentes

ABSTRACT

Movement is relatively invisible in literacy theory and pedagogy. There has been more recent scholarship on the body and embodiment, but less on connections between movements, body and literacy. In this article, we present the Community Arts Zone movement project and ways that the study opened up spaces for creativity, experimentation, and palpable identity mediation. Embodied space locates human experience within material and spatial forms. Drawing on Deleuze and Guattari's rhizomal ontology and Lefebvre's spatial theories, we examine how movement can be utilized to enliven pedagogy and to motivate people. During the research, classrooms, gymnasiums, and studio spaces became spaces that "the imagination seeks to change" by asking students to construct stories with their bodies. In the article, we present vignettes from our research study as telling instances showing the inherent strengths of movement as a form of literacy.

[A rhizome] is a map that is always detachable, connectable, reversable, modifiable, and has multiple entranceways and exits and its own lines of flight. (Deleuze & Guattari, 1987, p. 21)

Introduction

Like the rhizomes that Deleuze and Guattari (1983, 1987)) describe in their writings, this article shares moments when bodies move around spaces in a constant state of becoming without a middle or ending, always changing "in the middle". Applying the term rhizome within the reported research pushes our argument because there is a palpable sense of emergence implicit to Deleuze and Guattari's framing of rhizomes in *A Thousand Plateaus*. It is a useful term for the unfolding, in process nature of the movement work on display in this article.

The phrase "in the middle" captures an indeterminate quality of becoming. That is, at any given moment, a rhizome can move into what Deleuze and Guattari (1983, 1987) call a line of flight – a rupture in a rhizome which explodes into a line of flight (Deleuze & Guattari, 1983, p. 9). During our research together for the Community Arts Zone (CAZ) movement project, we witnessed rhizomes moving in different directions in space and every once in a while, lines of flight when the project came alive. Relating research reported in this article to Deleuze and Guattari's ontology, we focus on *the becoming of bodies* as ways of opening up imagined spaces (Lefebvre, 1974/1991) for young people. In the research, bodies exist in classrooms like rhizomes that expand spaces and ignite imaginings.

Movement is a form of literacy that is one of the more in-the-moment, spontaneous literacy practices. Movement exercises generated lines of flight and produced space. Drawing on more of Deleuze and Guattari's ontological theorizing of becoming (Deleuze & Guattari, 1987), we also apply line of flight to moments when movements converge into strong, relational sense making that students recognized. During the research, lines of flight became manifest when movements were in sync within groups of children and teenagers and when agentive practices were on display. Although the CAZ movement project was largely about bodies moving to music, in the end, it was space in physical and figurative ways that presided as the dominant theme. More specifically, movement work coupled with one or two other modalities like written narratives opened up pedagogic spaces in ways that we did not think possible. Classroom and gymnasium spaces noticeably changed when students engaged in movement exercises.

Bodily movement and gesture shape and reshape people by allowing both indivi-duals and groups to work in unison, or apart, to convey ideas, thoughts, and imaginings. Applying Lefebvre's (1974/1991) theories of space as produced and reproduced socially and sensorially, this article presents how students inscribe agency and think through a series of movement exercises and tableaux.

For the purposes of the article, we focus on analysing physical and spatial orchestra-tions to push for more work that places learners as embodied and emotional beings at the centre of analyses (Buchholz, 2015; Enriquez, Johnson, Kontovourki, & Mallozzi, 2015; Leander & Boldt, 2013; Lewis & Tierney, 2013; Medina & Perry, 2014). We begin the article by situating movement within a Deleuze and Guattari framework, we then examine the presiding theme of space and more specifically, opening up space when movement is introduced as a dominant channel of meaning making.

Generating lines of flight through movement and literacy

There has been some conflation of the terms movement and literacy into the phrase, movement literacy, by theorists who describe it as, "knowing *through* movement, knowing *about* movement, and knowing *because* of movement" (Kentel & Dobson, 2007, p. 150). Our definition of literacy within the CAZ research rests firmly on a belief that literacy involves several modes in play at once and these modes layer and are at times foregrounded and backgrounded during meaning making. Across all of the CAZ projects, literacy entails several modes working together and this presiding definition certainly pertains to the CAZ movement project. Indeed there is a growing tradition within literacy studies of research that focuses on the body and embodiment as part and parcel of literacy experiences (Enriquez et al., 2015; Leander & Boldt, 2013).

In our project, movement and thinking through the body were fundamental and connected strongly with other research studies that apply Deleuze and Guattari's (1987) call for understanding bodies as involved in social action and "as becoming rather than being" (Buchholz, 2015, p. 9). The appeal of applying a dimension of Deleuze and

Guattari's work is that rhizomes and lines of flight aptly capture a web of interactions between people, objects, sounds, spaces, other bodies that is beyond the rational and concrete. As the research in both schools progressed, it became clear that students involved in this project moved out of their habituated ways of being, knowing, and doing after doing movement work. Sitting in desks, standing for the national anthem, lining up for recess, these types of regulatory and habituated forms of movements were replaced with jumps, leaps, poses, and gesturing. The movements that students performed required expression, energy, nimbleness, and freedom. It was unbridled performativity within an environment that they were accustomed to view as narrow and didactic.

One of the best ways to illustrate unbridled performativity and a line of flight is to draw on moments during our research study as telling instances of practice. In the elementary school that we feature in the next section, there was a group of four boys who were often chatty, sometimes unruly and who clearly needed to move more. Glenys presented a movement exercise called verb chains where groups of four received a paragraph with verbs in boldface (see Figure 1) and they were asked to act out the verbs. Verb chains is an activity that Glenys teaches in her drama education work with undergraduates that involves people being the verb – "don't be the doer, be the done to" as she says. People take a verb like "beat" and give their own interpretation of what that is – existing within the verb as it were. When Glenys presented the activity, one group of boys in the corner of the classroom looked confused, larked about, and rolled their eyes. However, when this group of boys enacted each verb, we were surprised to find them serious and focused (even arguing) about interpretations of verbs like pump, circulate, and filter.

They asked Glenys for clarification and advice on verbs like "filter". They practised the verb chains several times. The verb chains allowed each boy to experiment with their bodies taking large, small, dramatic, rapid, and slow movements and working in sequence to move through each one. Each one did it in a different way and respected each other's interpretations, or at least they did not question or mock their interpretations. The movements were tubular like with one cascading into the next one in a fluid

Verbs- Circulatory System

The heart **beats.** Blood is **pumped** and **circulates** throughout the body. It **leaves** the heart through the arteries and **travels** and **flows** into smaller and smaller tubes until it **reaches** the blood vessels. Oxygen is **delivered** and **exchanged** with carbon dioxide. Blood **returns** from the blood vessels and **travels** through the veins to **return** to the heart. The lungs **filter** out the carbon dioxide and **oxygenate** the blood. This cycle **repeats** itself about once every minute.

Figure 1. Verb Chain movements.

way leading up to **oxygenate** as a culminating line of flight. There was a seriousness to their movement work and, at the same time, as a literacy practice it felt so natural and somatic.

Through their work on "performative pedagogy", Perry and Medina (2011) have shown how people can rethink and call into question conventional forms of meaning making by representing and thinking through bodies. Within our research, games as simple and enduring as tag became a way of uniting and melding together people who did not know each other into one space. The research relied heavily on what is performed and enacted as opposed to what is thought, meant, or practised. It was about collaborative practice and about bodies moving naturally through gut instinct and spontaneity.

The research created a new, different pedagogical space by asking students to complete movement exercises, sometimes to music, sometimes in silence. The research design involved visits to two schools observing teachers and students engaged in their everyday rites and practices and through scaffolding and movement strategies, a pedagogical space was transformed. To access initial perceptions and impressions about incorporating movement into the classroom, there were student and teacher interviews about their experiences with movement work and their thoughts about the relationship between movement and literacy. After initial visits and interviews, Glenys taught basic movement techniques – to ease teachers and students into using movement safely and with confidence – and presented the proposed assignments, while Jennifer documented what took place over the course of the 8 weeks. Throughout the research, Jennifer noted body movements, positions, musical responses and sound effects, gestures, degrees of engagement, drawings and images, words written and spoken, and gestures. Applying phenomenological methods, she focused on the essence of the experience (Merleau-Ponty, 1962). To do so, Jennifer took photos, drew pictures, and had brief conversations with student participants about how they experienced the movement work and later revisited these ideas during interviews.

The CAZ movement project rests firmly on Glenys's training with Jacques Lecoq, "one of [the theatre's] most imaginative, influential and pioneering thinkers and teachers" (Murray, 2003, p. 1) at his École Internationale de Théâtre Jacques Lecoq. Although we are not theorizing through Lecoq's framework, we signal his influence on Glenys's practice. Glenys believes that movement is a universal language that people lose when they enter the school years, despite the fact that, as Lecoq (2006) observes, "Children ... replay with their whole body those aspects of life in which they will be called on to participate. In this way, they learn about life and, little by little, take possession of it" (p. 1). Once a child enters formal schooling there is a dramatic change in how much movement they are allowed, and how much time they spend in desks, thereby ignoring what they have already intuitively come to know and rely on thus manifesting Lecoq's claim, "the body knowing before we know" how to move and think (Murray, 2003, p. 153). Throughout her career and during our project, Glenys incorporated elements of Lecoq's methods into her teaching, modifying movement exercises based on spaces, environments, and actions to provide "a method for analysing and evaluating ... [to expose the] "invisible poetry lying in the gaps "between words", [creating] "a playful tension between two very different ways of understanding or explaining" (Murray, 2003, p. 156) whatever subject was being explored. One specific technique for Lecoq movement is to extract active verbs from any event, sequence, process, or phrase in order to replicate the actions, attitudes, and ideas, using the ensuing verb chains to inspire close analysis and movement. For example, she would ask students to mime brushing their teeth then, to switch to full body movements to move like the toothpaste in their mouths. Glenys further explained this technique by describing a context such as a kitchen with all its attendant sounds and images and making them verb-rich activities (e.g. chop, sizzle, rattle) to invite certain kinds of movements. In other words, these verbs are metaphors to translate movement. As Lecoq (2001) describes it:

> We consider words as living organisms and thus we search for the "body of words". For this purpose we have to choose words which provide a real physical dynamic. Verbs lend themselves more readily to this ... each contains an action which nourishes the verb itself ... (p. 49).

Research methodology

The research study took place over 2 months during the winter and spring of the 2014 academic year. There was an elementary and secondary school involved which are described below. In terms of research methods, we took field notes, and Glenys took significant photographs and filmed students (purely for data analyses purposes). Even though the focus of the article is on rhizomatic patterns of production and the production of space, we feature field notes later that are tied, in some ways, to practice and meaning – but with production threaded throughout. We interviewed all of the teachers involved in the research and each teacher identified students who would be willing and interested in being interviewed at the end of the research. To analyse the data, we applied grounded theory and Wolcott's (2001) framework of interpretation, description, and analysis and we tended to privilege interpretation and analysis, especially examining our etic biases as modes of inquiry. We write from different perspectives, one a multimodal and literacy scholar and the other a movement expert and these biases are the filters through which we tell the story of the research study.[1]

Emic-etic data analyses

The study took place in two suburban, neighbouring cities, with distinct populations. The cities share demographics with long-standing white working-class families and more recent immigrants who have migrated to Canada. Framing social class is not clear-cut and often risks sounding deficit about communities and people. There are researchers who represent social class with a deft, sensitive touch (Collier, 2014; Hicks, 2002; Jones & Vagle, 2013). Falling back on such careful research, we have tried to sensitively frame social class in a manner that Code (2000) describes as "responsible inquiry that entails an effort to be 'true to' the everyday practices of knowing" (p. 217). The communities where CAZ took place are white, blue-collar towns with some unemployment over the years, primarily due to the collapse of the automotive industry and a lack of other employment opportunities. Children and teenagers involved in our research were from this population and as researchers we were often faced with our own lack of awareness about the everyday practices of our participants. In brief, we had false assumptions and in the process of uncovering everyday practices, we thought a great deal about responsible inquiry and what that actually means. One false assumption was that student participants had some experiences with extra-curricular arts activities outside of school and access to technologies and that these affordances were a part of our participants' lived experiences. During interview conversations, these assumptions were challenged and hearing their stories gave us the "rich back story" (Flewitt, 2011) that ethnographic perspectives can provide researchers and that clearly play a role in data analyses and our written accounts of the research. Although we both live in this community, false assumptions were made on our part and through the process of getting to know each other, we felt more confident about our responsible inquiry. One of the many enriching aspects of this research was the educators who were so in tune with their students everyday and who shared their stories and their lived realities. It is through these stories that we were able to add more depth and precision to the research.

As we wrote up the research, the concepts of emic and etic helped to tease out biases, blind spots, and assumptions during our data analyses. Through constructive feedback from reviewers, we went back to our data and created a table that featured emic facets and etic facets of the reported research. Ethnographers seek to acquire an emic or insider perspective by uncovering how people in a given culture think, feel, value, use language, and engage in particular roles and responsibilities (Bloome & Green, 2015). Ethnographers walk an often nebulous line between emic and etic or outsider perspectives as they move between their identities as an outsider/researcher with efforts to fit in and be an insider. We walked this line during the research and our reflexivity obviously informs findings in the article. To make the analyses more cohesive, we created a table with an emic facet column and an etic facet column with segments drawn from interviews, field notes, and photographs to illustrate our differentiation. Table 1 below shows an example of some emic versus etic thoughts.

What the emic-etic table did for our analyses is to make it more systematic and detailed in our thinking and it allowed us to look across the whole corpus of data to highlight when we imposed outsider views and how much they contrasted these with emic views – or simply to note the difference and make our biases more transparent. In the table, for example, views of the body spotlighted differences, even tensions between the two. As an insider to the school culture and with in-depth understandings about the diverse student body, Demi spoke from an emic perspective about students involved in the research. She talked about how different populations of students interpret movement. Drama students hoping to be actors or involved in media had a closer relationship, greater comfort and ease with movement and expression, whereas students in the technology education stream are less at ease and free with movement. Demi spoke from lived experiences with these students, appreciating that there are varied ways of viewing body work and how movement work is taken up. When Glenys spoke with Demi, they discussed how the mechanics of movement comes into play, with some students experimenting freely with movements while others feel hesitant or even incapable of doing certain movements.

An interesting finding in our study is that we anticipated body image would play a role in movement work with students, with students feeling self-conscious about their appearances. However, body image only arose with a small group of middle school girls

Table 1. Interpreting emic versus etic beliefs.

Emic facets	Etic facets
… Again it's just getting them to explore I think just what they can physically do with their bodies. Sometimes just getting them to think about how you move and how you can use different parts of your body to move and create things. Um and then I think the other complication might be that we do have kids that are actors and kids that are tech. They're willing, they're always willing to do stuff but the challenge will be to get them think outside of that box too.	David actually surprised me the most because he never struck me as someone who would participate at the level that he did. He is a very mathematically inclined person and always seemed a bit rigid and afraid of making a mistake. It was nice to see him open up and enjoy himself.
Interview with Glenys and Demi[2] (High School Teacher) May 2014	*Conversation between Jennifer and Language Teacher, June 2014*
… Movement exercises involved having your own body awareness like how can you stretch this way or you know just kind of exploring, not the everyday kind movement. Beyond the sort of more the abstract, thinking and thought and um. Just exploring your limitations to right so you may not think you can do something but how can you, you might not be able to do this, but how can you do this? Ya.	Such tight quarters in Kathy's room, hardly room enough to move around and desks and chairs everywhere. We are going to have to set up the room ahead of future sessions. A group of students had trouble completing activities in the corner of the room.
Conversation between Glenys and Demi	*Field note from 3 March 2014*

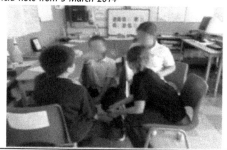

in the elementary school who did not want to be filmed or photographed. Body image therefore did not constrain movement work per se.

Research context

In terms of the specific contexts, the elementary school is a K–6 elementary school. The school is a faith-based school and we worked with an experienced grade 5 teacher. In our jointly written field notes, we agreed about our initial perceptions of the school:

> It is a public Catholic school and the teacher, Kathy, in her late thirties to early forties is committed to interactive, problem-solving teaching. We would describe her teaching as an inquiry-based teaching with structure added in to manage the large class. Glenys sees her as an inclusive educator – gently steering students to answers and stepping in when the need arises. The class is active with noise, but productive noise. When we met with Kathy a few weeks ago, she was concerned that we would find the class loud and a bit chaotic, but it was clear to us today that students love the environment and feel comfortable talking, interacting – even in a small, confined space. February 2013

When the research began, Kathy's programme dovetailed well with our movement research. What we agreed to do was to harness our movement work with her science unit on the circulatory and digestive systems. By the time we arrived for the movement sessions, the students and Kathy had created long lists of active verbs based on the circulatory or digestive system. Then, students in small groups (3–5), chose any five of the listed verbs for their group, and using their whole bodies, translated each "circulation- or digestion-based" verb into a "frozen picture" or tableau that were stages of the circulation or digestive process. For example, for digestion, some of the most popular verbs were: chew, swallow, disintegrate, squeeze, and expel. Students completed tableaux of digestive processes and they each created a movie trailer that charted out their tableaux before connecting the tableaux through movement.

The other context is a grade 9–12 high school, which is the second oldest high school in Ontario. The high school had more ethnic diversity than the elementary school and more of an entrepreneurial lens on curriculum (i.e. more of an emphasis on trades like hair dressing and auto mechanics). The research participants in the study were grade 12 ESL language learners teamed up with a smaller group of grade 12 advanced drama students. There were two teachers involved in the study; one was an ESL teacher with 18 years of experience and the other was a drama teacher with 8 years of experience and she is also a playwright. The ESL students came from such far-flung places as: Vietnam, Togo, Jordan, Iraq, Iran, China, the Philippines, and Korea. These language learners were reticent and concerned about the project because it was so unstructured and all of the movement work felt out of their comfort zone. The advanced drama students were more comfortable with the movement and tableau work. The 8-week movement assignment that they completed was based on the notion of a hero's journey that they would tell through a series of tableaux. Between each tableau there were also movement transitions – so there was therefore posed work and movement work existing in tandem. To complete tableaux, they had to consider what a journey is (e.g. a long, arduous journey like Odysseus on his long trip home to Ithaca, or a shorter, but no less meaningful journey, like falling in love and getting married). There were six groups that varied strongly in how they wanted to tell their journey story. By way of examples, one was the journey of two people falling in love and with family conflicts about the union and eventual resolution to the wedding day. Another was a grander journey with a young man going off to war and eventually returning home.

Space the imagination seeks to change

Lefebvre (1974/1991) argues that space constitutes human relations and practices. Social space where individuals live and practice their everyday lives can be viewed as a tool for thought and action. Lefebvre considers space in relation to macro constructs such as the ways in which capitalist regimes and nation states frame space as "owned" or as public or private and how these demarcations hegemonically leverage both power and status. This concept of framed or owned space emerged in both contexts when students engaged in quintessential schooling practices like sitting in a desk filling out a worksheet or reading texts silently at their desks. These normative, compliant types of activities imbued a heavy feeling to both settings. In contrast, the movement exercises that Glenys taught and that students enacted allowed for significant agentic variations or interpretations of stories or sequences of events such as a journey story or enacting the circulatory system. The negotiation of what these movements would look like within groups and the act of moving produced a social space that unfolded in multiple ways.

According to Lefebvre, there are rules and sanctions around the use of land or space that can reveal interplays of the powerful and the powerless. Thinking about Lefebvre's work on the production and reproduction of social spaces, it was clear to us then and now that even after a few weeks of working with the grade 5 and grade 12 students, classroom and gymnasium spaces shifted dramatically when students engaged in movement work. Lefebvre claims that spatial practices invite the social and the sensorial and these spatial practices produce and reproduce certain sorts of actions. During the research, "framing of the social" manifested themselves when students negotiated how to represent an idea through their bodies. When faced with a concept like food moving around in their stomachs or a soldier heading off to war, they would argue, negotiate, and debate about what movement best fits this message and how to orchestrate tableaux to express that action. In our field notes, we describe these moments as lines of flight that transformed spaces into imagined spaces.

Both pedagogic spaces resembled typical schooling spaces. The grade 5 context had desks in different groupings, a chalkboard, a white board, a teacher's desk, computers at the side of the room, and different posters, notices, and a Canadian flag. The physical space felt crowded, stuffy, and sometimes even claustrophobic. But, after spending time with Kathy (the teacher) and 28 students, the classroom changed transforming our initial impression of a cramped, messy room into a space with enthusiasm, excitement, and a sense of belonging. Indeed, the cramped feeling faded and in its place, there was a melding together of bodies with music. The grade 12 space was in a basement gym that had largesse but very little character – it was dark and long with pillars that separated out the space. In terms of its physicality, the gym was a big, empty room with chairs and tables on the sides of the room, and a low ceiling. There was a large chalkboard at the front and the room had dimmed, sombre lighting. Nevertheless, when bodies started to move and collide, the space became a lived space filled with energy and joy.

Drawing on spatial theory, Lefebvre (1974) starts from a belief that "spatial practice embraces production and reproduction, and the particular locations and spatial sets characteristic of each social formation" (p. 33). There is an acknowledgement in his work that people do things in physical spaces that elicit sensory responses. In his work, Lefebvre (1974) outlines three axes of space: "perceived space" of everyday life which signifies how our perceptions react to material worlds as they exist, influenced strongly by sensorial responses; "conceived space" as the particularities of spaces that can be concretized by individuals like cartographers making maps or architects drawing designs for rooms; and "the lived space" of the imagination which enlivens creativity and artistic interpretations and inspirations. As bodies moved around in a state of becoming much like Deleuze and Guattari's (1987) descriptions of rhizomes in A Thousand Plateaus, these axes of spaces moved in and out of each other. Lefebvre is clear that these three axes are always present, but sometimes foregrounded and backgrounded depending on the nature of the space.

Thinking about the grade 5 classroom as a perceived space filled with emotions, when we presented students with the movement project as a series of five tableaux that depict their science unit on the digestive system, they were reluctant, hesitant and their body language showed hesitation, but once they engaged in movement tasks with Glenys, their bodies softened and became what their teacher described as "nimble" and slowly, the perceived space transformed into a space of serious, thoughtful movement

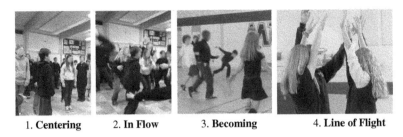

1. **Centering**   2. **In Flow**   3. **Becoming**   4. **Line of Flight**

Figure 2. Rhizomes in spaces.

practice. As a conceived space, the classroom that from the outset appeared crowded, dark, messy, chaotic, and full of 28 bodies in a small, confined space, opened up and felt more expansive. Certainly after 5 weeks of movement tasks with Glenys and once they had completed their short films of five tableaux, they moved into a large gymnasium and it was at this point that the lived space came to fruition.

Moving into the school's gymnasium, two filmmakers filmed the grade 5 students for the CAZ documentary and that was when the imagined space came alive. In Figure 2, we represent a steady movement across two spaces from a centring activity in their classroom to the realization of their movement work into a line of flight in the gymnasium. It is a line of flight because the four students came together into a structure that they built and that drew them together in a relational, semiotic chain. It represents a *line of flight* because their rhizomal movements of becoming were realized in the moment and there was a palpable impression of sense making and then they moved onto another set of movements. For the centring exercise, students closed their eyes, listened to their breath, and felt their sense of weight transfer as they gently moved their bodies forward and backward – in that moment, the classroom space expanded for them. There was not a rowdy, silly feel to their movement work, but instead, a patient, measured feel to their movements that we capture in the second image as "In Flow". In the third and fourth images, "Becoming" and "Line of Flight", we adopt Deleuze and Guattari (1987) phrasing to depict how students seemed to experience a flow and becoming leading to a crescendo that we think of as a line of flight or rupture that then moved quickly into other rhizomes of movements.

There was no attempt to be structured, but there was an effort to be calm and to focus. There was a democracy, or at least an effort to be democratic and to listen. There needed to be a consensus when they reached their line of flight.

Vignettes as instances of practice

To illustrate our theorizing of the CAZ movement project, we profile what we call instances of practice or moments in field notes when spaces transformed and when students moved in and out of states of becoming (Deleuze & Guattari, 1987). The first vignette took place when we first introduced movement exercises into the grade 5 classroom. Kathy, the teacher, was on hand to help manage the group while we demonstrated the movement work.

Instance of practice 1: opening up spaces

The number of students in the class took us aback. The desks took up a lot of space. There were many students with different issues such as attention issues and a girl who was a selective mute. They were used to going off on their own. It took them a while to come into movement. They were fine if they had the teacher right there. The movement work underlined the issues with focus problems for the students. It took a while to calm them down – they went crazy and could not focus on the task. We both felt strongly that the space would not work.

Kathy was the suggested teacher. She is self-effacing, shy, and more comfortable with kids than adults. She had an uncanny ability to know when to release them and when to let them in. Her classroom was a comforting place, all of the time. You would think that her classroom was utterly chaotic, but it wasn't. She was brilliant at getting the best out of each child.

The lesson of the day involved making bridges of straws, popsicle sticks, masking tape, and they used a hair dryer to test their constructed bridge's efficiency, weight, and durability. It was a mini-lesson that exemplified her entire pedagogy – kids can do it their own way – they had to come up with a product and answers and they had to come up with the answers collectively.

The mood and space shifted when Glenys did centring. Glenys told students to listen and feel how all of the muscles are working as you go over the soles of your feet. Find your centre and the internal listening that shut them down. Once we did that, the whole mood shifted. 7 February 2013

Kathy's open pedagogy involved using blocks of time to work with materials and solve problems. To contrast the lively nature of the bridge construction, Glenys quieted the mind with the centring activity. Laughing at first, once children closed their eyes there was an almost immediate stillness that filled the room. Students worked at their own pace and Kathy was attuned to each student's rhythm. In other words, Kathy tended to foreground Lefebvre's first axis by having students view their classroom as a perceived space and by encouraging students to think through their senses. Though the actual space was cramped, Kathy masterfully made students experience the space as open, lively, and with room for freedom. Watching her class at work, there were clusters of bodies congregating in different parts of the cramped space, content and focused and working through tasks at their own pace. But, the moment described above involved noise, some rowdiness, and excitement, especially when they tested their bridges in front of the class. The students imagined the space beyond any physical or material constraints.

Instance of practice #2: follow the leader

The other vignette happened with the high school group during an introductory exercise called *magnetic attraction* where there is a leader and a follower – each person using a different body part to lead or to follow (e.g. the leader uses right elbow as point of direction, follower uses left shoulder with an 8-inch separation between shoulder and elbow).

Then, the music of Raphael Gato Fuentes (Glenys's husband who is a composer) created a mood-based atmosphere. So, something slow and inspirational versus slow and suspenseful or something spooky and dark to set the mood and put bodies in motion. The trick is that it is not popular music – there are no connotations – no connections – it was not visually mediated so it won't co-op your thoughts. It is also architectural – students can respond physically and emotionally. They can position themselves like buildings on a street or like statues. There was an interposing of music and body parts in space. The music picks you up and carries you along. Movement helps with focus – "it fills in the emptiness and the silence." 15 March 2013

On this occasion, Glenys inducted students into a movement, embodied mindset. Students required time and gentle encouragement to get over their inhibitions and simply play with music and movement. Glenys presented an activity that allowed students to play with body relations and with positioning bodies in different ways to transmit a message. Moving beyond words to direct action and then adding in sound pushed students to think about concepts in very different ways.

What surprised both of us, once again, is that these teenagers were comfortable facing each other and engaging in movement exercises that entailed close proxemics. We imagined laughter and blushing, but instead we encountered serious faces concentrating on deliberate movements. The mix of language learners and advanced drama students situated themselves all around the expansive gymnasium and mimicked movements that were open-textured and filled with interpretative possibilities as they quickly transitioned into another mirrored movement. This is where the coupling of Deleuze and Guattari's framework with Lefebvre's notions on the production of space work so well together – they place great emphasis on "coming in being" (Lefebvre, 1974, p. 67). There was a *becoming* (Deleuze & Guattari, 1987) with a coming into being in the gymnasium as a conceived space that moved into an imagined space through music and movement. The emergence of selves in a social space led to various representations. Connecting to Lecoq, the emergence and representation continuum in the act of becoming hints at Lecoq's "the body knowing before we know".

Instance of practice 3: the Greek chorus

Glenys and Demi (the teacher) used music to make movement fluid and it worked well. The beauty of Raphael Gato Fuentes's music is that it does not have lyrics and combines softer songs with active ones. The music noticeably loosened inhibitions.

After the Greek chorus exercise, students then worked on their journey that followed five phases: 1) Awareness; 2) Departure; 3) Obstacle; 4) Fulfillment; and, 5) Return. Students were asked to write down phrases that made them think of each phase. I worked with a few groups and again the language learners had some difficulty with vocabulary. In particular, the group of boys – Simon and his friends – struggled with ways of capturing awareness. I too had difficulty starting with awareness as the beginning of the journey. Consulting with Glenys and Demi, we changed it to a reason why one goes on a journey. I spoke at length with a teenager who moved from the Philippines to Ontario and how difficult it was for him to adjust to Canadian life. Then, I spoke with a teenager from China who moved to the area to learn English and she had a very difficult time with her host family and her parents had to come from China to live with her here. The story reminded me of how brave they are to come on their own to a new country because they are still teenagers after all.

After working on their journey stories, students got into pairs (deliberately pairing language learners with native speakers) to do a marionette activity. Glenys modeled the activity with a student showing how to pretend that they are attached to strings and the strings control movements. 3 May 2013

Abandoning fears and self-consciousness, the teenagers became inventors and their embodied actions conveyed certain sorts of meanings, whose "translations" seemed to embody echoes of their first language. By that we mean English language learners could express with their bodies what their second language, English, could not convey, but that their first languages did. As Lecoq (2001) remarks: "According to the language being used, words will not all have the same relation to the body" (p. 49). The Greek chorus ignited a series of lines of flight by the students working together. The concept of crafting a story through poses and then movement transitions bound groups and helped them move through a series of becomings. Figure 3 depicts a particularly memorable line of flight when a shy language student from the Middle East came out of his shell and became Odysseus in their tableaux of an arduous journey.

Instance of practice 4: seen/unseen

Moving back to the grade 5 classroom, there were some students who did not enjoy the movement work. More specifically, there was a cluster of girls and boys who often told one of us, "I do not want to appear in the documentary and please do not make me do my tableaux in front of the group". We respected their wishes. A revelation for us came when we suspected that a selective mute girl WOULD BE SHY AND WITHDRAWN asserted herself into the most lively and engaged triad of girls to do movement work. Once again, our false assumptions were that selective mute translates into shyness and a disinterest in physical work in groups. We were definitely wrong about this and this comes out strongly in the following field note:

> There is a day during the document filming that I recall so vividly. It was in Kathy's grade 5 classroom when Glenys asked students to plan out and orchestrate five tableaux of the digestive system, that would then have "appropriate" mood music added and that the Four Grounds guys would film. I remember the resistance that we had from a cluster of boys and girls. Glenys and I were worried that the boys wouldn't take the activity seriously, or, that they would be reduced to uncontrollable laughter, or, that they would be bored. I remember one student in particular who came out of her shell when filming started. Natalie (pseudonym) had been diagnosed as a "selective mute" at the beginning of the school year and she had hardly spoken a sentence since then. Kathy allowed her time and space to

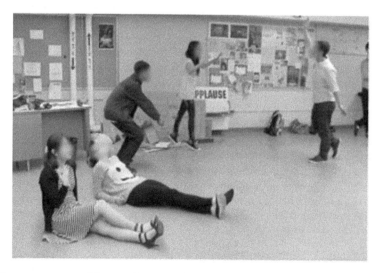

Figure 3. Teenagers engaged in movement work.

work gently into things. To our surprise, with a little coaxing, she joined the movement activities – in group and pairs work – although at first, she did not add to the verbal negotiating. However, over the next few weeks, when asked questions during the movement sessions by Kathy, Glenys, or me, she began to answer very quietly, in short phrases. This change translated well into her movement work, so that by the end of the sessions she was adding longer phrases and short, but complete sentences to her group's planning conversations, and despite a high level of noise from groups talking simultaneously in "preparation mode", she was speaking clearly and loudly enough for her small group to hear her. 15 April 2013.

When we probed Kathy more about Natalie and about particular students, Kathy kept going back to the basis of her teaching – "it is all about listening – building that foundation with them where they feel like they can talk". There was something about the somatic, embodied practices that we completed that allowed Natalie to be seen by her peers in ways that were not deficit. Spoken communication was at arm's length from her and it freed her to make meaning in alternative ways.

From limp flowers to nimble movers

A secret to the success of the CAZ movement project rests on the distance that it created between rhetoric like "grade-appropriate development" or "emergent reading to fluent reading" versus somatic, natural expression. The research was at arm's length from top-down, value-added, neoliberal kinds of agendas, and on a simple level, the project allowed two groups of students to move around and be nimble. On a deeper level, the project constructed a new imagined space for children and teenagers to express themselves and to rupture into lines of flight. McDermott (2005) once said that "language, literacy, and learning are about being in the world. They do not have to be about a rush to teaching" (p. 123). In our modest study, the only teaching that happened was a movement expert sharing techniques and exercises.

At the beginning of the research, when we interviewed Kathy about her grade 5 students she shared that they "could be like limp flowers" during the school day in her classroom. She said, "these kids live difficult lives at times and …. I want to create a creative, fun space for them". Both of these reflections struck a chord for us as we finished up our data collection – we returned to her sentiments as we wrote up this article. During student interviews and brief conversations, we had windows into the realities of these students' lives. Realizing our etic perspectives were imposed on this culture, we relied heavily on Kathy and Demi and their emic, rich understandings about the lives of their students. Our aim in this article has been twofold: one is to show how a pedagogic space opened up, figuratively speaking, when students express themselves through their bodies; the second aim is more couched and hidden, which is to amplify or animate the need for a far bigger, nuanced, rhizomatic picture of literacy. Of course, you could very well ask, where is literacy in this article? Like other articles in this special issue, it is everywhere – it is in bodies, in voices, in silence, and in gazes. Literacy is profoundly human and natural and as such, has so much to do with the natural meaning making that we witnessed throughout the project.

Returning to Kathy's observations, at the beginning of the research we saw limp flowers, but we most certainly saw the opposite – excited, energetic, vibrant children in motion. In their cramped classroom or in the expanse of their gymnasium, it really did not matter, they moved in deliberate, thoughtful ways and not in chaos and disorder (which is one's first impression). Put to music and film in the CAZ documentary, their movements looked orchestrated and elegant. It truly was a space where the imagination changed. Movement as a literacy or a form of meaning making (which is how we prefer to view literacy) became an area of deep connection for these learners.

Notes

1. The research study has received ethical clearance from the Brock University Research Ethics Board (File # 13–016 Rowsell), the District School Board of Niagara, and the Niagara Catholic District School Board.
2. Pseudonyms are used throughout to protect the identity of participants and contexts.

Disclosure statement

No potential conflict of interest was reported by the authors.

Funding

This work was supported by the Social Sciences and Humanities Research Council of Canada [Grant number 430-2013-1025].

References

Bloome, D., & Green, J. (2015). The social and linguistic turns in studying language and literacy. In J. Rowsell & K. Pahl (Eds.), *The Routledge handbook of literacy studies* (pp. 19–34). London, UK: Routledge.

Buchholz, B. A. (2015). Drama as serious (and not so serious) business: Critical play, generative, conflicts, and moving bodies in a 1:1 classroom. *Language Arts, 93*(1), 7–24.

Code, L. (2000). Naming, naturalizing, normalizing: "The child" as fact and artefact. In P. H. Miller & E. K. Scolnick (Eds.), *Toward a feminist developmental psychology* (pp. 215–237). New York, NY: Routledge.

Collier, D. (2014). "I'm just trying to be tough, okay?": Masculine performances of everyday practices. *Journal of Early Childhood Literacy, 15*(2), 203–226. doi:10.1177/1468798414533561

Deleuze, G., & Guattari, F. (1983). *On the line*. Boston, MA: The MIT Press.

Deleuze, G., & Guattari, F. 1987. *A thousand plateaus: Capitalism and schizophrenia*. (B. Massumi, Trans.). Minneapolis, MN: University of Minneapolis Press.

Enriquez, G., Johnson, E., Kontovourki, S., & Mallozzi, C. A. (Eds.). (2015). *Literacies, learning, and the body: Putting theory and research into pedagogical practice*. New York, NY: Routledge.

Flewitt, R. (2011). Bringing ethnography to a multimodal investigation of early literacy in a digital age. *Qualitative Research, 11*(3), 293–310. doi:10.1177/1468794111399838

Hicks, D. (2002). *Reading lives: Working-class children and literacy and learning*. New York, NY: Teachers College Press.

Jones, S., & Vagle, M. (2013). Living contradictions and working for change: Toward a theory of social class-sensitive pedagogy. *Educational Researcher, 42*(3), 129–141. doi:10.3102/0013189X13481381

Kentel, J. A., & Dobson, T. M. (2007). Beyond myopic visions of education: Revisiting movement literacy. *Physical Education and Sport Pedagogy, 12*(2), 145–162. doi:10.1080/17408980701282027

Leander, K. M., & Boldt, G. M. (2013). Rereading "a pedagogy of multiliteracies": Bodies, texts, and emergence. *Journal of Literacy Research, 45*(1), 22–46. doi:10.1177/1086296X12468587

Lecoq, J. (2001). *The moving body: Teaching creative theatre*. New York, NY: Routledge.

Lecoq, J. 2006. *Theatre of movement and gesture*. (D. Bradby, Trans.). London, UK: Routledge.

Lefebvre, H. 1974. *The production of space* (1sted.). (D. Nicholson-Smith, Trans.). London, UK: Blackwell Publishing.

Lefebvre, H. 1991. *The production of space* (2nded.). (D. Nicholson-Smith, Trans.). Oxford, UK: Wiley-Blackwell.

Lewis, C., & Tierney, J. D. (2013). Mobilizing emotion in an urban classroom: Producing identities and transforming signs in a race-related discussion. *Linguistics and Education, 23*, 289–304. doi:10.1016/j.linged.2013.03.003

McDermott, R. (2005). "An entry into further language": Contra mystification by language hierarchies. In T. C. McCarthy (Ed.), *Language, literacy and power in schooling* (pp. 111–124). Mahwah, NJ: Erlbaum.

Medina, C. L., & Perry, M. (2014). Texts, affects, and relations in cultural performance. In P. Albers, T. Holbrook, & A. S. Flint (Eds.), *New methods in literacy research* (pp. 115–132). New York, NY: Routledge.

Merleau-Ponty, M. 1962. *Phenomenology of perception*. (C. Smith, Trans.). New York, NY: Humanities Press.

Murray, S. (2003). *Jacques Lecoq*. London, UK: Routledge.

Perry, M., & Medina, C. (2011). Embodiment and performance in pedagogy research: Investigating the possibility of the body in curriculum experience. *Journal of Curriculum Theorizing, 27*(3), 62–75.

Wolcott, H. (2001). *Writing up qualitative research* (2nd ed.). Newbury Park, CA: Sage Publications.

Embracing the unknown in community arts zone visual arts

Jennifer Rowsell and Peter Vietgen

ABSTRACT

Telling stories through photographs is certainly not a new or novel concept; however, thinking about image-making as a way of unknowing what we currently know is quite different from traditional approaches to photography. Built on an existing conceptual framework, writings on unknowing, we apply unknowing as a guiding method and heuristic to understand what a group of young people are trying to say and reimagine through the act of image-making. Research reported in this article from the Community Arts Zone visual arts project features a series of photograph projects across high school contexts where students created a Cindy Sherman-style conceptual photograph with an artist statement. The researchers engaged in a process of unknowing to interpret the photographs where they read through the visuals and engaged with modes in play and with observational fieldnotes about participants to draw out implications for such work for literacy teaching and learning.

Introduction

This is an article about how young people perform identity in photographs as a form of unknowing (Vasudevan, 2011). Using a mode of questioning, we interpret photographs that young people produced over 6 weeks to embrace a reimagining of what teaching and learning can be like when frameworks are loosened and permitted to be slack, free from the constraints and measures of more regimented schooling life. Adopting a method of *unknowing* encouraged by Vasudevan (2011), we ask questions about student-produced photographs, inviting the stories that students tell through photographs to be contemplated, and we pause to appreciate the exercise of allowing young people to be provocative, imaginative, and disruptive in school spaces without imposing rules or frameworks on their work.

Within literacy studies and related fields, there is a recognition of the power of the image as a knowledge-producing medium for young people (Hull & Nelson, 2005, 2009; Kinloch, 2009; Sefton-Green, 2013; Vasudevan, 2011). At the heart of our project is an interest in the image as an improvisational medium that provides freedom to question and that allows for different forms of identity performance. Image-making, like writing, is how we come to know the world and our relationship to/with it. Unknowing as a form of inquiry into images allows us as researchers to think about what young people pay attention to. Divided into five parts, the article begins with an explanation of the process of unknowing (Vasudevan, 2011), then we profile visual discourse analysis (VDA) as a form of unknowing and questioning stories in photographs, followed by a presentation of the Community Arts Zone (CAZ) visual arts research and case studies of student photographs, ending with a return to unknowing as a heuristic for arts-based approaches to meaning-making.

A process of unknowing

In order to loosen more rigid ways of viewing literacy teaching and learning, in the reported research we approach ideas, concepts, and archetypes that students fore-ground in photographs through what Vasudevan calls *unknowing*. Unknowing involves a series of such questions as: "How do we pay attention?" or "Where do our imaginations live?" or "How do we step outside – or enable, prepare, and support ourselves to conceive beyond – the scope of our imaginations?" (Vasudevan, 2011, p. 1158). As Vasudevan notes, "The ways in which we perceive – the world, one another, the situations we encounter – are not straightforward or simple" (p. 1159). Add to this the fact that we bring our own worlds and subjectivities into the analyses. Even though we spoke with research participants about their image-making, the process of unknowing is so unfettered, so fluid, so provisional that one can never know defini-tively what is being said by the image-maker of the photograph. One can appreciate angles, colours, costumes, and poses and have a general sense of a photograph, but one cannot know in a deep sense the imaginings that led to producing an image. In this paper, the research participants are engaged in the unknowing process. Nevertheless, questioning goes some way in accessing the ethos and message of the final product. As Vasudevan eloquently expresses it, "at any given moment, questions about 'what is' rather than 'what isn't' can lead to new horizons of 'what might be'" (p. 1160).

There is something more humane about complicating any form of meaning-making – whether it is an essay, an image, or a film. Vasudevan talks about how "seeing with feeling, creatively, imaginatively, may perhaps lead to the founding of institutions of education and educational inquiry as welcoming sites of being" (p. 1162). In the photo-graphs featured later there are 'straightforward' messages like a girl dancing or a young man hoisting a car like a superhero and there are more complex, layered images depicting eating disorders, body image issues, and lost cultural heritage, but who is to say that one is straightforward or complex and who can impose an interpretation? More to the point, viewing and contemplating the photographs should entail a process of deliberate and deliberative reflection. As Arendt (1968) argued, "storytelling reveals meaning without committing the error of defining it" (p. 105). Young people featured later were certainly telling us stories, but who are we to state what those stories are? They are not our stories to tell. Yes, we can describe images; yes, we can state what we think the images depict; and yes, we can speculate on stories; but, we cannot tell the stories ourselves. As researchers, there is a tendency to drift into what is comfortable and familiar, but as Vasudevan acknowledges, "how do we prevent ourselves from slipping into casual determinism?" (p. 1168). Together we have found it productive, even generative, to unknow what we know.

Images, unknowing, and the everyday

One of our motivating factors for examining how young people take conceptual photographs is the ubiquity of contemporary image-making that is part of the every day. You cannot venture too far without seeing someone taking, repurposing, or remixing a photograph, yet within literacy studies, we still do not have a robust language for how to think and communicate through photographs. Take Figure 1, which is a photograph by a 15-year old playing with images on Snapchat. Snapchat works on a logic of filters whereby an image is taken and then, upon viewing it, it instantly disappears. The whole point of the exercise involves capturing a mood, thought, effect, and impact to communicate to another person. This young woman sent the Snapchat to her Mum to be fun and whimsical, but also to say – I am fine and with my friends. But, who is to say that is exactly what she is saying. These fluid, dynamic, and deeply embodied interactions display a brand of imagination, thinking, and creativity that is tied up with experiencing a moment in time and playing with that experience. I am here now wearing doggy ears and a doggy nose – where are you? Or, ha-ha, guess where I am? Rather than using words to communicate these moments, people opt for visuals that pass and fade out. These fluid, playful practices recall what Vasudevan calls "dwelling in an imaginative space" (p. 1157). Within this process, senses and aesthetics are central – "aesthetics reference arts ability to be responsive to or pleasing to the senses" (Harste, 2014, p. 96). Our response to the world relies so heavily on our senses. Observation and play with art and multimodality can transform and call into question thoughts and

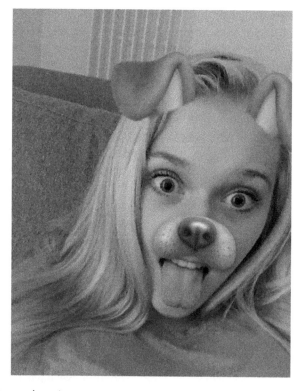

Figure 1. Snapchat as unknowing.

beliefs. White (2011) says that "art renders back to us not simply what we see, but how we react to what we see and what we know as a consequence of that seeing" (p. 3). Seeing, touching, listening, speaking, and moving, there are expectations for texts today to not only include a number of modes at once, but even more so, to actively elicit reactions and senses in dynamic, fluid, often entangled ways. There seems to be a constant ebb and flow of making and unmaking – seeing design/production as a form of knowledge. There is such an ambiguity about Snapchat filters that allow for unknowing through identity play and creative semiotic banter between people. Ambiguity is a key dimension to Snapchat and part and parcel of the logic of the social media outlet.

Talking to young people about image-making, we differentiated three types of images that they talk about: disappearing images; transitional images; and fixed images. Ephemeral, disappearing images are ones that you take to engage, interact, and socialize with others, often through social media, with apps like Snapchat or Instagram. Transitional images connect across spaces and places that are both vast and small, but their central purpose is to share information about yourself to signal agency. Facebook and professional sites like LinkedIn are examples of image-driven genres that use images for more immediate news about self, and these types of photos and images are transitional in nature, giving viewers a picture of someone's life and lived experiences in the moment. In this article, we showcase a third category of images, *fixed images*, which are statements that can be enduring and that can hang on walls as a reminder of a moment, a memory, a story, or even a thought. We believe that fixed images are a neglected image genre in education, and they represent an opportunity for educators to concentrate on the art and craft of image-making.

CAZ visual arts research background

As one of the five CAZ projects in southern Ontario, CAZ visual arts consisted of photography projects in three high schools in neighbouring cities. To conduct the research, we drew on the photographic style of Cindy Sherman who is famous for her conceptual photographs of archetypes and concepts, and she is both the photographer and the photographed in her shots. We worked closely with high school teachers and students over 6 weeks in three secondary school sites until students completed their own conceptual photographs and attended an exhibition of their work at a local art gallery.

As noted, Cindy Sherman portrays ideas, personas, archetypes, and identities in her photographs, and she is both the participant in the photograph and the photographer. In 2012, the Museum of Modern Art (MoMA) profiled Cindy Sherman's work of over 40 years in an exhibition and on the MoMA website about the exhibition they describe how Sherman foregrounds the eclectic nature of her photographs:

> Whether portraying a career girl, a blond bombshell, a fashion victim, a clown, or a society lady of a certain age, for over thirty-five years this relentlessly adventurous artist has created an eloquent and provocative body of work that resonates deeply in our visual culture. (MoMa, 2012)

The appeal of Cindy Sherman's work lies in her capacity to disrupt stereotypes and archetypes and to engage in identity work through photographic and design techniques. Sherman's work is conceptual in nature, offering broader commentaries about societal issues like the varied roles and depictions of women. Cindy Sherman tells visual stories that are not predictable and that are not without contestations and tensions. We found that the young people in our research responded strongly to Cindy Sherman's work and to the idea of representing parts of their lives such as indigeneity, homophobia, and bulimia or to alter egos like a superhero or Marilyn Monroe and John F. Kennedy. Accompanying the photographs were artist statements that extended their stories and gave students a forum to further express why they chose particular figures to represent and express themselves in some way.

The CAZ visual arts research design entailed an account of context combined with ways in which students performed their identities in photographs. As well, as with the entire CAZ research study, there was an overarching multimodal orientation to meaning-making wherein two or more modes were always in play during project work. As opposed to focusing on process or product, we preferred to think of the Being Cindy Sherman assignment as questioning, journeying, and experimenting to find a photographic style. We conducted interviews with three case study students in each high school as well as taking fieldnotes during observations and hands-on work with students. The students were chosen by their teacher. All teachers involved in the research were interviewed, and their perspectives underpin our analyses.

Research contexts

The projects took place in three secondary schools in neighbouring cities. Millsford High School (pseudonyms throughout) is one of the oldest high schools in Canada with vaulted ceilings and turrets; the school is a landmark in the small city. Students who attend this high school are predominately from working-class families with some racial, ethnic, and religious diversity. The high school has a strong technical education programme, and students are mostly college bound or intend to enter trades like mechanics, media jobs, and plumbing. There were 10 student participants involved in the research, all of whom have physical, mental, and developmental disabilities. Stokewood High School is in another small city, and the high school is well known for having famous film and media alumnae. With this cinematic and media pedigree, the school has a huge wing entirely devoted to media studies and to the media arts. There were 12 students involved in the research, the majority of whom were from indigenous backgrounds from different bands in the area. Our third school, Morton Heights Secondary School, is a 10 minute drive from Stokewood High School. Morton Heights is a school with a high academic presence, and the majority of the students attend university after graduation. Our class at Morton Secondary School consisted of 24 senior high school visual arts students. As a result, there was a diverse range of young people engaged in the research and these divergent perspectives were thrown into relief in the photographs.

In terms of our roles, Peter is both a visual arts scholar and a professional photographer, and these roles circulated within data collection and analyses. Jennifer comes from a media and publishing background that strongly informed her data collection and analyses. For some time, Jennifer has excavated visuals and artefacts for visible traces of identities and social contexts. As Gee (2005) says, meanings in multimodal texts are "assembled on the spot" (p. 94), and Jennifer concentrates on how materials and modes are assembled and designed and she couples this perspective with an account of the social map of multimodal work (i.e. identities of producers and the nature of the contexts where texts are produced and how these forces get embedded in texts). By social map, Jennifer refers to the meaning maker or meaning makers involved in the design and production of the multimodal text. The social map includes the context of production, the actors involved in its production, the materialities drawn upon to produce it, and the practices used to make the text.

Research design

The research entailed observational fieldnotes, multimodal analyses of photographs, and exit interviews with nine research participants. We interviewed nine students selected by their teachers as ideal interview participants across the three schools. Although both of us had conversations with the participants over the course of 12 visits to the schools and we attempted to document the culture of the schools, the research cannot be considered an ethnography in the formal sense, but rather what we think of as touches of ethnography in our efforts to get to know participants, educators, and the school cultures. Beyond what is revealed in the photographs, our knowledge about student lives and backgrounds was fairly limited, and the focus of our data analyses is on how students mediated their identities and/or expressed their interests, beliefs, and what we came to regard as their ways of unknowing what they know *through* images.

Applying VDA

To interpret student photographs, we apply Albers' (2014) interpretation of visual discourse analysis (VDA) complemented by student interviews that we conducted at the end of the study. According to Albers, VDA combines the strengths of semiotics as an explanatory framework for visual texts that are "a structure of messages within which are embedded social conventions and/or perceptions … which also present discourse communities to which the visual textmaker identifies" (Albers, 2014, p. 87). Conflating visual analyses with discursive approaches to texts, Albers uncovers larger constructs, critical engagement with ideas and conventions, beliefs, thoughts, and emotions communicated in visual texts by combining an account of visual elements with linguistic elements. The combined strength of these two elements makes the interpretation richer because students not only produced photographs, but also they wrote artist statements about each photograph. Peter maintained that photographs must have an artist statement to give participants another vehicle to describe their productions. Peter agrees with Albers' point that there is a limited view of texts if seen from one interpretive optic, combining two or a cluster of modalities offers communication a greater complexity that it needs and deserves.

During our fieldwork, we therefore applied similar types of questions as Albers, for instance: How is language used to communicate (use of technique, design, colour, etc.)? How do viewers respond to the context of the text? Why these design choices and not others? What is revealed about the text-maker through the image (attention to discourses and systems of meaning that underpin the visual text)? And how does art act as a force on viewers to encourage particular actions or beliefs? This line of questioning comes from Albers' interrogation of texts through VDA (Albers, 2014, p. 88), and it certainly helped us to excavate visual narratives. As well, there are the larger questions implicit to a process of unknowing such as, "How do we step outside – or enable, prepare, and support ourselves to conceive beyond – the scope of our imaginations?" (Vasudevan, 2011, p. 1158).

Armed with Albers' and Vasudevan's questions and provocations, we spent 6 weeks with the different groups of participants, beginning with presentations of Cindy Sherman's work, to brainstorming their image ideas, to gathering artefacts, materials, and visual effects, to executing their shots, to choosing their featured photograph, to writing their artist statements, and finally, to curating a museum space. Figure 2 is a photograph of the museum space before people arrived and speeches were given. We became well acquainted with participants and their processes and pathways into multi-modal work (Kress, 1997).

Following Albers' techniques and methods, we sat together to visually scan all of the finished products and chose telling examples of students' privileging of different discourses, ideologies, and beliefs with their photographic compositions. Initially, we sat side-by-side and looked at the photographs, then Peter selected photographs that stood out to him as a photographer, and we discussed them and then further refined which ones we could focus on for the article. Applying Albers' visual discourse process, we then talked about photographs holistically in terms of semantics; then we read structures within each text, paying particular attention to photographic techniques that we taught them and ones that they acquired through osmosis or their own experience with image-making – given the number of photographs that they take and share in a day.

Finally, after coding interview data through open coding or "first phase coding" (Saldana, 2013) which entailed detailed line-by-line analyses, we generated as many codes as possible and then matched them up with our visual analyses based on Albers' framework to graphic and syntactic information. After this process, we interpreted objects, the placement of objects, colours used, vectors, lighting, and the orientation of the image (Albers, 2014, pp. 88–89). Peter adopted this form of analysis given his

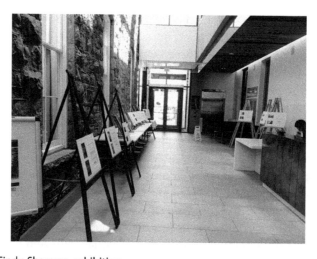

Figure 2. Being Cindy Sherman exhibition.

years of experience as a photographer, and Jennifer tended to focus more on discourses, meanings, and identity-laden practices. Finally, Albers applied Koch's concept of "recurrent pictorial elements" (cited in Sonesson, 1988, p. 38) as elements that cut across texts. Some of these elements appeared in photographs whilst others appeared in artist's statements. Later, we highlight some of the recurrent elements within photographs.

Behind the lens

There is a complexity to thinking behind a camera lens that for a novice feels a bit hapless without some instruction and practice. The photography teacher in one of the three high schools described his philosophy of teaching photographic methods by focusing on life lessons:

> When teaching photography, I focus on life lessons and what is going on in the world and let them go from there … I try to get teenagers to function a little more normally as adults in society and to understand the big picture through photography. (Jonathon,[1] 13 April, 2015)

Working alongside students, we found it best to watch participants decide on an idea, research it, experiment and use trial and error to figure out the style, impact, and aesthetic, and Peter would step in with technical tips and strategies. Combining instincts with technical instruction that they acquired from Jonathon and Peter and through conversations with each other, researchers and teachers, each participant brought their own experiences and dispositions into the image-making process to tell a particular story. As noted earlier, some of these statements had to do with weighty issues and topics like alcoholism, substance abuse, and racism, and some were lighter like displaying pure joy, or a favourite TV show or media icon – it did not really matter, what stood out as substantial and meaningful were the choices that they made and subjectivities invoked to do so. As Jonathon noted during our interview, so many of the teens started the project with apathy about school, either not showing up or when they did being dismissive and saying that "they are not creative" and this changed slightly after they produced their photographs, but it did reinforce a general malaise about school.

Behind the lens, there was a falling-off of inhibitions and constraints and students embraced an unknowing as

> an act of dwelling in the imaginative space between declarative acts of knowing and not knowing; an invitation to wrest our modes of inquiry and our beings away from the clutches of finite definitions of knowledge and instead rest our endeavours in the beauty of myriad ways of knowing. (Vasudevan, 2011, p. 1157)

During the CAZ visual arts project, time and again, we documented students journeying into visual stories, and what intrigued us is how they translated their visual stories into written narratives in their artist statements. As Jonathon reflected on the process, he argued that once they committed to the project, they were absorbed – from experimenting with different shots, to seeing the photo become a reality on paper, printing, matting, and hanging it. It was not a perfect process. There were struggles along the way such as students' inabilities to adhere to photographic rules and conventions like the rule of thirds which did not come naturally to many of them. According to Jonathon, "our brains want to put images in the centre." Pushing students to shoot a little off-centre was difficult as was having them think seriously about angles, lighting, and proximity. Peter, Jonathon, and other visual arts teachers with whom we worked talked students through these techniques and design rules and principles, and some students applied them while other students had to experiment with them before they found the right shot.

The overall goal of CAZ visual arts rested on changing student perspectives through photography. As Jonathon said, I hope to "change the way that they look at the world that they live in through photographs." The fact that younger generations take photographs more than ever and that there is an abiding passion for visualizing and documenting lives in social media fed into many of our discussions with participants about what they saw and how they could conceptually frame what they saw to express or articulate their feelings and beliefs. So many of our students spent their time documenting their lives visually on Snapchat and Instagram, but there was a qualitative difference between their transitional photos and the fixed ones that they produced for the project.

Being Cindy Sherman: image analysis

Two exemplary photographs from Morton Heights Secondary School are featured below to illustrate alternative pathways into visual work. One depicts an issue in a young woman's life that concerns body image and specifically eating disorders. The other is a tribute to gothic worlds and, in particular, the popular show, *The Addams Family*, and the posed couple depict Pugsley and Wednesday Addams. The photographs are different in nature with interesting compositional effects.

In the Addams Family image (Figure 3), both students knew exactly what they wanted to present – characters in the show; accurate costumes; posed, serious expressions; and an opulent yet foreboding background that invites viewers to look up at the characters. Their artist statement is quite simple – "Listen to the children of the night; What sweet music they make." – Dracula. Clearly, they wanted to tell an alternative story about themselves and they wanted to embody a darker version of their lives. Speaking with the two young people, they were clear at the time that they did not want the photograph to be light and kitschy, but instead elegant and somber. They achieve this effect by appearing in front of a heritage building in their town that has been there for well over 100 years. They are looking down at the viewer with expressionless faces.

Thinking about Albers (2014) line of questions: language simply communicated their message about the darker side of childhood; there is a macabre feel to looking up at the couple; the visual and written narrative reveals an exacting, even mischievous side of both participants; and as far as actions and beliefs, the photographers call on the viewer not to underestimate the figures presented as merely popular culture icons, but to see them as sinister and substantial figures. There is a sense of informality to the photograph, as if you would see these two individuals on the street and know that they are different, and perhaps sinister but not terrifying by any means. Applying Vasudevan, what is in the photo is a historic, heritage building and two figures in the archway looking down at the viewer, but what is not there is a clear connection to the media text or to the story behind their interest in the Addams family. There are several other unknowns within the image. As a visual composition, it is incredibly effective at drawing a viewer into the photo.

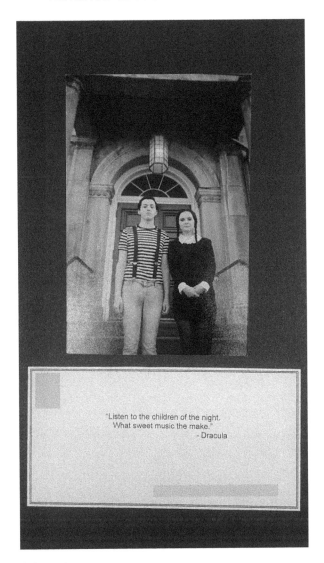

"Listen to the children of the night.
What sweet music the make."
- Dracula

Figure 3. Children of the night.

With the Scales image (Figure 4), the participant and photographer opted for a stark, striking image about eating disorders jarring the viewer into thinking about it through a visual narrative focusing on a young girl hanging over a toilet presumably vomiting surrounded by a scale, pills, food, and towels. The written narrative accompanying the photograph beautifully states the point: "Scales are essential to fish in the sea; but not essential to human beings." Returning to Albers (2014) interpretative framework: words and images do not match with words describing scales on fish and the scales that people use to weigh themselves. Focusing on discourses of body image and body dysmorphia; art acts as a force by compelling the viewer to look down on the image and to feel constrained, maybe even constricted by the space. It is a photo filled with suggestions to a theme, but it is hard to say what the young woman is precisely saying – about herself, about the issue, and about the image more generally. The image-maker

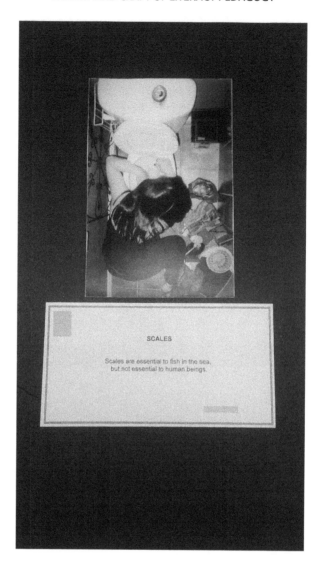

Figure 4. Scales.

does not state clearly what she is saying about bulimia or even naming it, but her image is rife with suggestions.

As shared earlier, at Stokewood High School, we worked with a group of indigenous students from First Nation bands in the area. The indigenous students live in a city beside the US border. Students at Stokewood High School gravitated naturally to their own backgrounds and heritage, without any prompting; in essence, they wanted to tell stories about their cultures and tribes. In Figure 5, Cameron proudly holds his Mom's painting, and in the backdrop the viewer can see a friend who is smiling and sitting on a sofa. The statement matched up with the visual talks about his Mom's painting as expressing pride about being indigenous and his Mom's efforts and talents and as someone who provides constant guidance. In the second photograph, Cameron faces the viewer with determination and sternness – "This is our land ... damn it! This is our

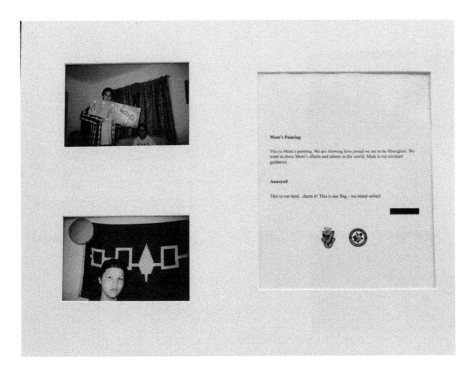

Figure 5. This is our land ... damn it!.

flag – we stand united!" The coupling of the photographs is Janus-faced with joy flanked against anger and loss. Compositionally viewers are drawn into the objects: the bright pink painting replete with symbols and the Iroquois Confederacy flag, which was at one time the original Canadian flag. Both are representing culture, language, and heritage in quite different ways. What the painting says about the photographer is his absolute pride in his Band and his Mom. Cameron faces the viewer with an expression that says I am not here to please you viewer, I am here to pay tribute to my Band and my family. There is a reliance on artefacts in these two images to speak for Cameron, and they are relational artefacts connected with his family.

Thinking about Albers (2014) framework, words and visuals equally exert power and steadfast resolution to the viewer. The photograph acts as a force on viewers by encouraging them to acknowledge the Iroquois flag. Here I am, acknowledge me and, more importantly, acknowledge the history that has been obfuscated, rendered silent, even taken away. The image reveals Cameron's conflicted sense of loss and deep allegiance and commitment. It is a photo montage that makes a strong statement about land rights and forgotten histories. This is declarative in the photographs, but there are dimensions of the images that we cannot venture to know and this is where the unknowing process comes in.

Flank Cameron's photographs against Anya's images with a different feel and ethos to them, yet they express many of the same messages that Cameron foregrounds by considering her deep roots with her culture and people. In the first photograph (Figure 6), Anya sits in front of an indigenous image of a multicoloured turtle. For Anishinaabe peoples, the turtle is a spirit animal representing wisdom and for Anya,

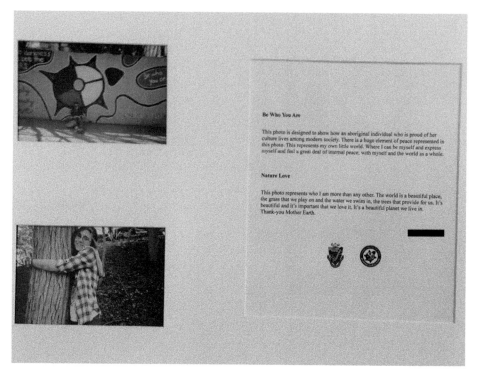

Figure 6. Thank you Mother Earth.

this is the precise location where she sits and for her, it imbues a sense of peace and comfort. It is a place where she can express herself and feel at home. In terms of Vasudevan and unknowing, it is a place where her imagination lives and where she can journey in her thoughts with ease, without judgement. In the next photo, Anya embraces a tree connecting strongly with Mother Earth and with the beauty of nature. Anya looks overjoyed to be there and to be expressing her deep connections with the earth. Anya discussed both images with us and indeed struggled with what she would write (as most of the students did).

As strong as Anya's photographs are, especially the one of her hugging a tree, what sits with both of us are her artist statements. Beside the photo of her in nature she says,

> This photo represents who I am more than any other. The world is a beautiful place, the grass that we play on and the water we swim in, the trees that provide for us. It's beautiful and it's important that we love it. It's a beautiful planet we live in. Thank you Mother Earth.

Asking, to what do we give attention, in the artist statement is quite clear – pay attention to the earth and to nature. Compositionally, colours jump out of the first photograph of a turtle, and positioning is a strong technique in the second photograph with Anya hugging the tree on the left side of the photo with a larger open leafy space beside her. The texture of the tree is so vivid that you feel like you can reach over and touch it. In Albers' terms, art acts as a powerful signifier of Anya's heritage.

Anya's photograph emphasizes the living of culture as opposed to the doing of culture that Street talks about when he theorizes culture as a verb (Street, 1993). As a text-maker, Anya was clear about wanting to inscribe her love of nature and her people, and this comes out strongly in both her photograph and artist statement. During our interview with Anya, she claims that a driving force of the image is "our mother earth heartbeat and it represents nature as religion." She maintains that her pictures go together in a dialogue because "one shows where I go to be with my culture and the other shows what I am with my culture." As Vasudevan articulates it, nature "enables, prepares, and supports" her "to conceive beyond the scope of our imaginations" (p. 1158).

Moving to Millsford High School in a neighbouring city, we worked with a smaller group of students with a range of disabilities. What threads through our experiences at Millsford are strong emotions and a greater enthusiasm about the process. This can be seen clearly in Amy's photograph in Figure 7, with her wearing a blond wig striking a theatrical pose singing into a microphone with the impactful t-shirt that has LOVE emblazoned on the front. Amy was so clear and focused about the photograph – she knew that she wanted to "look pretty" and she was determined to sing Justin Bieber's song, "Baby." She described to Peter how much she loves the Cheetah Girls and how she

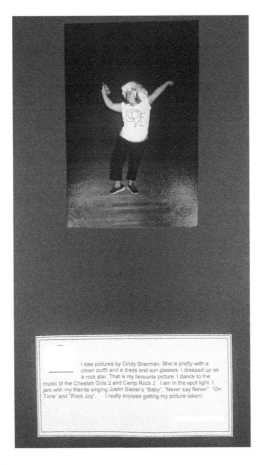

Figure 7. Love and joy.

dances to songs in the movies and this informed her decision for this particular visual. There is unmistakable joy in the image. It has energy and it encapsulates so well Amy's verve and bon vivant character. Amy tells the viewer that she loves music, dancing, and feeling free. As an act or statement, the photograph centres on the story that Amy wants to tell the viewer and not one that is imposed upon her.

As a final image from the Millsford research, we present Scott's photograph (Figure 8). Scott was not sure about what he wanted to depict for his Cindy Sherman photograph. In the end, he had an epiphany as we did a tour of different parts of the high school which has a mechanic's studio, a full chef's kitchen, a hairdressing suite, and a welding studio. Once Scott saw the mechanic's studio, he knew that he wanted to depict a superhero with superhuman strength. Having created many superheroes with different names from Massive Saver to Red Cardinal to Spider Teen Lady Ninja, Scott insisted that he would portray Massive Saver in a

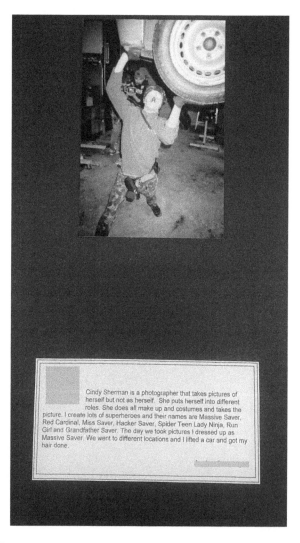

Cindy Sherman is a photographer that takes pictures of herself but not as herself. She puts herself into different roles. She does all make up and costumes and takes the picture. I create lots of superheroes and their names are Massive Saver, Red Cardinal, Miss Saver, Hacker Saver, Spider Teen Lady Ninja, Run Girl and Grandfather Saver. The day we took pictures I dressed up as Massive Saver. We went to different locations and I lifted a car and got my hair done.

Figure 8. Superhero.

strong, dramatic pose in the midst of imminent danger – a car about to fall on his head. Scott wanted to exude immense power and strength, the ability to hoist up a car with one hand. The art acts as an alternative story of his own reality – contrasting a meek, somewhat shy young man with someone who has superhuman strength and fearlessness and indeed the written narrative reinforces this too. A key point when thinking about both Amy and Scott is that they struggle with their writing, and this assignment gave them an opportunity to try another medium and mode of expression to talk and express and for people to listen.

Why is image-making agentive? How does unknowing help?

Throughout the article, we have insisted that photographs are agentive and thinking across images seen in the article, *What precisely is agentive?* To us, a literacy scholar and photographer-visual arts scholar, it is the ambiguity, emergence, and the evanescence of images that makes them so agentive. The image-maker and receiver bring their own stories to bear on their interpretation and in doing so, they invoke agency. Stories like images cannot be absolute because they are always told by someone with their own set of subjectivities. It could be argued that it is tougher to pin down an image – especially conceptual ones in the styles of photographers like Cindy Sherman. By their very nature, conceptual photographs invite interrogative work to figure out the mystery and ambiguity which invites agentive responses. This is where unknowing as a method of inquiry can help. With image readings and viewings, people bring histories, biases, past visual experiences, and this unfolding of layers while taking or viewing images gives a partial view and unknowing allows, as much as is possible, a shedding of ideologically and socially produced lenses, to try to see things differently. Images cannot be absolute because the meanings are agentively, socially, culturally produced by the image-maker and viewers equally bring subjectivities to their viewing.

Returning to the language of description at the beginning of the article, disappearing images; transitional images; and fixed images, all of these genres of images tell stories which are sometimes real, sometimes imagined, and sometimes a combination of the two. Disappearing photographs are abbreviated moments of expression to connect or laugh or emote; transitional images speak across groups and create affinities; and the fixed images that you saw in the last section make statements – but, they all tell stories. These are dynamic stories in that they can move and change and serve as dialogic pieces (think about the logic of Snapchat or Instagram), but it seems clear that they are agentive in that they are a way of telling people something in some way which is always an interpretation.

Anya, Amy, Scott, and Cameron told stories about who they are or want to be in the world. Imposing an unknowing lens on images and artist statements opens up, to some extent and certainly more can be done, a looser, less-restricted space. It was unbridled, it was creative and playful, and it was deeply agentive. There are many more questions that can be asked of them that will open up and reimagine more worlds.

Thinking about Vasudevan's presiding questions, *what do we pay attention to?*, often the business of education pays attention to the concrete and to the measurable. The trouble is that the concrete and the measurable sit within out-moded and out-dated conceptions of learning which are qualitatively different today. It is no wonder that young people often seem disengaged and apathetic about school. It is not necessarily the fault of teachers because as

Jonathon illustrates, they understand the lives of their students and they do all they can to motivate them. With three distinct groups of teenagers serving as our study participants, not all three maintained a steady continuity of momentum to bring the research project to completion. There were ups and downs with identifying what image to take, with gathering artefacts, with finding contexts in which to take photos. There were also obstacles such as using a disposable camera or processing photos and realizing that they do not appear as the photographer had hoped. One thing, though, that was clear for all of the participants, was the sense of pride and accomplishment they felt at the exhibition openings of their final photographs at the respective galleries. On those evenings, they felt they had a voice. Their photographs, accompanied by their artist statements, served as a vehicle to express loud and clear, who they were and what their views were on the world around them.

In thinking about what we pay attention to, we both agree that we pay attention to the teachers and the young people in our research. They were fundamental and we learned more from them than they learned from us. Conversations during the process and catching glimpses of image inspirations and story-boarding, and hearing peer-to-peer exchanges fed our desire for more emic perspectives on image-making. Questions remain and knowing stories in any full sense remains hazy, but what seemed evident was how images drove perception and imagination.

Disclosure statement

No potential conflict of interest was reported by the authors.

Funding

This work was supported by the Social Sciences and Humanities Research Council of Canada [grant number 430-2013-1025].

Note

1. We use pseudonyms to protect the identities of teachers and students involved in the research study.

References

Arendt, H. (1968). *Men in dark times*. Orlando, FL: Harcourt.

Albers, P. (2014). Visual discourse analysis. In P. Albers, T. Holbrook, & A. S. Flint (Eds.), *New methods of literacy research* (pp. 85–98). New York, NY: Routledge.

Gee, J. P. (2005). *An introduction to discourse analysis: Theory and method* (2nd ed.). Abingdon, UK: Routledge.

Harste, J. C. (2014). Transmediation: What art affords our understanding of literacy. Paper Presented at the Literacy Research Association Annual Conference in Dallas, Texas. Retrieved from http://jeromeharste.com/recent-publications/

Hull, G., & Nelson, M. (2005). Locating the semiotic power of multimodality. *Written Communication, 22*(2), 224–261. doi:10.1177/0741088304274170

Hull, G., & Nelson, M. E. (2009). Literacy, media, and morality: Making the case for an aesthetic turn. In M. Prinsloo & M. Baynham (Eds.), *The future of literacy studies* (pp. 199–228). London, UK: Palgrave Macmillan.

Kinloch, V. (2009). *Harlem on our minds*. New York, NY: Teachers College Press.

Kress, G. (1997). *Before writing: Rethinking the paths to literacy*. New York, NY: Routledge Press.

MoMa. (2012). Cindy Sherman: About the exhibition. Retrieved from http://www.moma.org/interactives/exhibitions/2012/cindysherman/about-the-exhibition/

Saldana, J. (2013). *The coding manual for qualitative researchers*. London, UK: Sage.

Sefton-Green, J. (2013). *Learning at not-school*. Cambridge, MA: MIT Press.

Sonesson, G. (1988). *Methods and models in pictorial semiotics* (Report 3 from the Semiotics Project). Lund, Sweden: Lund University.

Street, B. V. (1993). Culture is a verb: Anthropological aspects of language and cultural process. In D. Graddol, L. Thompson, & M. Byram (Eds.), *Language and culture* (pp. 23–43). Clevedon, UK: British Association of Applied Linguistics.

Vasudevan, L. (2011). An invitation to unknowing. *Teachers College Record, 113*(6), 1154–1174.

White, K. (2011). *101 things to learn in art school*. Cambridge, MA: MIT Press.

Imperfect/I'm perfect: bodies/embodiment in post-secondary and elementary settings

Kari-Lynn Winters and Mary Code

ABSTRACT

Using researched perspectives of bodies and embodiment, along-side dramatic structures, where bodies are foregrounded, this article looks closely at bodies and embodiment inside of school settings. Specifically, it investigates a community in Southern Ontario and the perceived, affective, relational, and critical ways that study participants story their identities about their bodies. Findings suggest that body image itself (i.e. how youth perceive their bodies) and embodiment (i.e. how youth use their bodies for communication and learning) are vital but sometimes invisible topics in today's school settings, where bodies are continually interpreted, admired, shamed, moved, rejected, and positioned. Though drama and other subjects like the arts focus on embodied ways of knowing and offer unique opportunities for learning, they can also hold unique challenges in school settings.

During a drama workshop about body image, Sofie (an elementary student), who has just volunteered, steps into the role of the designer at the mannequin factory. She stands tall, despite the fact that she has her hand in front of her face, covering her mouth. Here, the researcher is in role as well, as the boss of the factory.

Researcher (in role of factory foreman):	And what's your job then?
Sofie:	Designer of poses. I make the...um... positions of the...
Researcher:	of the mannequin?
Sofie:	Yes.
Researcher:	Ok, what do you need?
Sofie:	My mannequins are perfect – like super perfect!
Researcher:	Good.
Sofie:	But...why do you want them perfect anyway?
Researcher (confused):	Because I want to sell my company's clothes and...
Sofie:	Well, I think you'll sell more clothes if you make your mannequins realistic...

Others:	So people take it seriously.
Researcher:	But I need perfect mannequins!
Sofie:	Perfect is different for different people.
Others:	Yeah. Like…she's right. Make different shaped mannequins. That actually look like the shapes of different people, real people…then more people will buy them.

As part of an international Social Sciences and Humanities Research Council (SSHRC)-funded research project, which took place in four different communities worldwide, the authors of this smaller study used playbuilding and dramatic structures (where bodies are foregrounded) to investigate and explore notions of body image and embodiment within school settings. Specifically, this smaller study paid attention to the ways bodies are semiotic and socio-critical texts (representations) that are read by others, as well as sensed and affective modes of creation (tools) that produce, inscribe, demonstrate, and animate information (Grushka, 2011; Perry & Medina, 2015). Sometimes the ways that bodies are inscribed and the ways that bodies inscribe are not always aligned. This can be problematic in schools and universities when students are asked to present, report, move, and perform in front of others. Not only are teachers/professors putting students in the line of others' gazes and positioning them in certain ways, but also because the student's intentions can become muddled (i.e. their embodied authorship can be mis-read or misinterpreted by others).

The vignette above begins to demonstrate the ways bodies are perceived, admired, rejected, and positioned within a school setting. Here, using a Mantle of the Expert approach (Heathcote & Bolton, 1995), elementary students were put into the roles of experts and were asked to design "perfect mannequins". In this moment, Sofie, a 5th grader, stands up to the foreman of the factory, refuting the idea that there is such a thing as a "perfect" body. As she speaks, she covers a scar on her face with her left hand. While she indicates with her posture (standing tall) that she is confident, her gestures (covering her face) suggest otherwise – leaving room for others to misread her body language.

Later, after the workshop, the researchers asked Sofie's teacher to describe Sofie. The teacher stated that Sofie was "mostly non-verbal and shy". She went on to say that Sofie often covers her mouth and gazes downwards because she has a cleft palette scar. The teacher then stated, "I was nervous when you asked Sofie the question, 'Ok, what do you need?' because Sofie is typically so shy". The teacher expressed that she did not know if that question would distress Sophie or put her on the spot. Oppositely, the teacher said that she had never seen Sofie so confident. She went on to say that she rarely discusses body image or social issues with her students because she does not "want to deal with" or "is afraid of the reactions". Weeks following the study, the teacher stated that though it is challenging to communicate about underlying social issues such as body image in schools, she felt it was "vital". She expressed an interest in using the arts as a way of addressing these issues.

Context of the study

The goal of the bigger, SSHRC-funded, international Community Arts Zone (CAZ) project was to explore the arts within different contexts, paying particular attention to the ways that people interact with art, use various modes for meaning-making, and collaborate within various communities. More specifically, the bigger project connects broader notions of literacy, creativity, embodiment, affect, critical thinking, and situated community practice. In this article we focus on one of the seven arts-based study sites (other sites focused on music, mural-making, building structures, youth theatre, photography/visual arts, and movement). This smaller project happened within the Niagara region in Southern Ontario. We feel that our smaller study contributes to the other seven CAZ research studies in four important ways. First, it expands notions of multimodal, situated, and critical literacies, demonstrating how theories of embodiment have the potential to inform notions of authorship and the arts in school settings (Barton, Hamilton, & Ivanic, 2000; Kress, 2010; Pahl & Rowsell, 2012; Winters, 2010). Second, this study focuses on various modes of meaning-making (e.g. writing, playbuilding, acting, singing), yet illustrates that in practice all authorship is multimodal, lived (or improvised), and participatory (Siegel, Kontovourki, Schmier, & Enriquez, 2008; Stein, 2008; Winters & Vratulis, 2013). Third, the study portrays elementary and university students engaging in active pedagogies within their own communities, showing that the arts and literacy are not as separate as school systems sometimes make them out to be (Winters, 2010). Fourth, this study suggests the sensitivity with which teachers may need to have/be aware of when using the arts within different community contexts.

The smaller study took place over a ten-month period in Southern Ontario from 2013 to 2014. Data were collected from 783 study participants, including community members, elementary school teachers, post-secondary students, and elementary students. The majority of these participants were Caucasian and middle class.

It is the hope of the authors that this article will add to a growing conversation about bodies and embodiment within post-secondary and elementary school settings, specifically assembling four perspectives: (1) body image; (2) affect; (3) relational authorship of the body; and (4) discursive embodied positions. Our research questions align with these perspectives. (1) What observations do post-secondary and elementary students make regarding bodies/body images during arts-based practices, including how do students feel about their bodies? (2) How do students use their bodies to communicate with (relate to, react to, align with, sense, reject) and position themselves and others within these school settings? (3) How might a better understanding of bodies/embodiment within school settings inform/shape pedagogical practices?

This study included three phases:

(1) Community stories were collected from local organizations (e.g. those dedicated to weight loss, community recreation, writing craft, and wellness). This invitation allowed participants' agency to share their experiences in relation to the research topic.

(2) All of these stories – along with additional resources, such as picture books and novels – were gathered and brought to fifteen post-secondary undergraduate theatre students. Working with the instructor of the course, students planned, scripted, and rehearsed a 45-minute play about body image over eight weeks, meeting once a week for three hours each session. Using a playbuilding approach, the play itself combined musical theatre, comedy sketches, soundscapes, digital collage, dance, voice montage, improvisation, and choral reading. This play was

then presented in two school boards (eight schools in total) to over 780 students, many of whom were interviewed or asked to participate in focus groups.

(3) The author of this paper and her research assistant returned to present drama in education workshops using Dorothy Heathcote's Mantle of the Expert pedagogical framework (Heathcote & Bolton, 1995) to all of the elementary students in all eight schools.

Qualitative data sources included stories from the local community, videoed scenes and work samples, scene breakdowns and blocking charts, director's notes, interviews with students and teachers, photography, focus groups, and artifacts.

Next, these data were coded by theme and then transcribed. Based on the focus of this article, three vignettes (as well as the introductory vignette) were selected. These three vignettes, as with the one above, were chosen because: they look closely at struggles that the students encountered with their own body image or with embodiment in school settings, they relate to the theories that are being foregrounded in this article, and they offer different perspectives from all three phases of the study.

The authors chose to analyze and represent the chosen vignettes using different embodied drama structures: (1) alter-ego, (2) mirrors, and (3) hot seating. This arts-based approach is an attempt to put theory into action, exploring the felt and evolving experiences of bodies, including knowledge that complexly and simultaneously engages in the semiotic, the relational, the affective, and the critical – knowledge that "defies language" (Gallagher, 2015, p. xv).

Situated methodology and situating the researchers

As a part of situating the research, particularly within lived experiences of embodiment, it is important to acknowledge the background experiences and subject positions of the researchers themselves. Just as the researchers are also a part of the situated contexts, they are thus a part of the study results. Unpacking the unseen assumptions, motivations, and ideas of the researchers cannot only broaden the scope of the study, but also can deepen understandings of how the study participants move, act, respond, and share their experiences, positions, and knowledge.

To this end, the authors, Kari-Lynn and Mary brought a broad array of background experiences to this project. As a playwright, performer, storyteller, teacher of elementary school children, and an associate professor to teacher candidates in the fields of literacy and arts education, Kari-Lynn's focus in this project varied throughout the three phases. In the first phase, she elicited stories from various communities. Her intention was to encourage other writers and storytellers to take part. Some of these writers asked Kari-Lynn to read over or edit their contributions before sharing. In Phase two, she collaborated with the instructor of the university theatre course to assist in building the play with the post-secondary students. Kari-Lynn used her background experience and post-secondary education to take on the roles of workshop facilitator, co-director, production co-manager, and dramaturge. Finally, in the third stage of the research project, Kari-Lynn went into schools with her research assistant, Mary, with the intent to both facilitate a Mantle of the Expert workshop for the students and also to explore and challenge their notions of body image and media. Kari-Lynn and Mary drew upon their acting training and their backgrounds in teaching to take on various roles: workshop facilitators, drama in education teachers, interviewers, etc.

Mary pulled from her background experiences as a researcher, student of drama in education, and lifelong member of the arts community. She came to the elementary schools with the intention of exploring students' perceptions of bodies and body image. She wanted this exploration to be centered on a facilitation of meaningful drama-based activities that could be used as a catalyst for dialogue with students that would recognize their voices and help them to celebrate "imperfect" bodily features.

Both researchers positioned themselves as guests within the schools, who were informed and practiced in theatre performance, in teaching students, and promoting arts-based pedagogies. The schools, including the staff and students, viewed Kari-Lynn and Mary as knowledgeable experts in drama and as scholars, and introduced them as such.

The subject positions that both authors assumed and assigned play an important part in the larger assemblages that were authored in the study as their values, beliefs, prior experiences, and assumptions frame not only the positions of others, but also inter-weave with the affective and embodied realities of the study. In other words, the materialities of the context, the situated practices and structured routines, and the spaces themselves, as well as the actions of all of the participants involved (including the researchers) play an important role in this study, but also in the methodology that was used to develop and understand this study.

Entry points for research on bodies and embodiment

While exploring several research perspectives on embodiment, Perry and Medina (2011) acknowledge that "bodies are both a representation of self (a 'text') as well as a mode of creation in progress (a 'tool')" (p. 63). This idea sounds simple, but when one thinks about bodies and embodiment, it is complex. For not only is the body a fleshed moving vehicle by which humans sense/experience the world (biological), it is also: a sign for the representation and inscription of meaning (semiotic); an encapsulation of thoughts and affect (philosophical and psychological); a part of a larger relational entity such as a community (post-structural; affective); a pathway of engagement into sociocultural, historical, and political practice (culturally performed; socially theorized; critical, femin-ist); a discourse of power (Foucaultian); an interacting entity on a shared plane of influence (post-humanist); and so forth (Perry & Medina, 2015). Additionally, bodies are "media-tized", represented in magazines and commercials in order to be adorned, adored, shamed, gazed at, and envied (body image). Moreover, bodies are also schooled within institutions – moved, physically and discursively positioned, even trained. Indeed, with so many entry points for research, scholarly work on bodies and embodiment has the potential to be quite complex. In fact, scholars have only begun to scratch the surface of what can be claimed about bodies within schooled settings.

Due to the fact that this field is so vast, we the authors wanted to focus on an assemblage of four entry points for representing and analyzing the data: (1) body image; (2) affect; (3) relational embodiments/authorship of the body; and (4) discursive embodied positions. The research perspectives and vignettes we chose for this article do not go into detail about several important theories – critical race, phenomenology, psychology of bodies, cultural performance, humanistic, Marxist, critical feminism, or disability studies – for example. This is not because we found these paradigms less influential or significant, but rather because we only had so much space in this article to represent our ideas.

Body image: bodies as perfection

The elementary children in the vignette above were initially trying to create the "perfect" body (mannequin), inadvertently comparing their own bodies to a perceived "ideal". During this process, they created body maps which demonstrated both their confidences and their insecurities about their own bodies. Ninety-three percent of these body maps demonstrated dissatisfaction in some form or another.

Research demonstrates that there is a growing dissatisfaction with bodies in our society (Cash & Pruzinsky, 2002; Woodcock, 2010). Bodies are too flabby, too skinny, too hairy, too short, and so forth. Influenced by social media and other body-focused texts (e.g. songs, movies, avatar games, fitness and weight loss propaganda, body modification, advertisements and commercials), people are paying more attention than ever before to the ways that their bodies compare with others (Smolak & Thompson, 2009). Perhaps social media and digital technologies are partly to blame for this ongoing problem? Indeed, the word "selfie" only recently (within the last 10 years) became a familiar term and was added to established dictionaries such as the Oxford Dictionary.

Regardless of the cause, media internalization is a growing concern in both school and out-of-school contexts, playing with the ways that youth and even children gaze upon others and also see themselves. Smolak and Thompson's (2009) book on body image suggests that since 2001 there has been an explosion of research to demonstrate that many young girls and boys struggle with body image, including weight-related problems. Murnen, Smolak, and Mills' (2003) research study with grade-school children demonstrates that youth exposed to media not only experienced more body dissatisfaction, but also had the potential to demonstrate body rejection responses, which in some cases lead to future eating problems and mental health concerns. Some scholars discuss a de-personalization process that can happen, where a person experiences one's body as disconnected from oneself (Jacobson, Hall, Anderson, & Willingham, 2016). Thus, just as a person witnesses the bodies of others as separate from his/her own, he/she might also view his/her own body in that way too, disconnecting from how one's body is both feeling and functioning.

Social comparison in adolescence plays a significant role in self-perception as children strive to be leaner and more attractive. Furthermore, research shows that girls whose body shapes were further from "ideal" reported greater dissatisfaction with their bodies (Smolak, Levine, & Thompson, 2001).

Ideals about bodies not only come from images/media that are witnessed, but also from body perceptions that are formed inside of social relationships and that occur within situated contexts – between one's body and its social environment (Piran & Teall, 2012). For example, one study by Janet Liechty and her colleagues (Liechty & Lee, 2013) explored how children were able to express their positive and negative perceptions of body image, even as young as preschool. The scholars went on to say that family beliefs, behaviors, and everyday practices influence young children's awareness on body image development, even though parents said they did nothing to influence their children. This suggests that media internalization and sub-conscious embodied communication patterns are occurring regardless of conscious attention. Beyond family structures, body image constructions can also be shaped by cultural influences, and even religious beliefs (Jacobson et al., 2016).

Affect: bodies as sense-able

Often in schools, bodies are thought of as the fleshy containers that move our brains from place to place/class to class, merely vehicles that transport us. Yet bodies have enormous potential to know as well – to sense and to make sense of our environments. Bodies not only feel physical sensations, but also construct knowledge about one's environment and infer the feelings of others. In other words, embodiment is sensed (and SENSE-able) as bodies physically perceive the contexts around them, coming "into productive relationship[s] with thought and language as our sentience asserts itself" (Gallagher, 2015, p. xiii).

This knowledge guides humans in situated contexts and shape identities. Feelings and sensed impulses continually interplay with thoughts. They are part of our histories and cultures, and they play a role in shaping our present and our futures. Emotions are experienced and lived through bodies as well as voice, and they are also brought to life and circulated through public culture (Ahmed, 2004).

In the vignette above, the others support Sofie as a collective body. They sense her urgency and intentions, and insist that nobody (no body) is perfect. Furthermore, perfection is different for everybody (every body). Through dramatically informed structures and participatory, hands-on activities they come to feel a collective and emerging doubt about perfect bodies.

Drawing on the work of scholars like Hochchild (1983) and Sara Ahmed (2004), Kathleen Gallagher (2015) cultivates the notion of the effects/affect of emotion, noting that emotions do not reside merely within individual bodies, but also within larger bodies of communities. "…[E]motions are not held within individual bodies, but are rather produced as effects of bodies and emotions in relations" (p. xiv).

Relational authorship: bodies as communication

Communication, the imparting or receiving of information, is a relational and layered process, especially when bodies, voices, and cultural/material resources are examined together within socially situated contexts. Silent meanings are authored through gestures, facial expressions, postures, and gazes. These actions are felt by others, seen by others, read and interpreted by others. In this way, bodies are always authoring and social relationships are always being authored. For example, Sofie's teacher felt that her student was shy and vulnerable because of the way she hides her scar, despite the fact that Sofie was the one person who had the confidence to stand up to her foreman.

Understanding the body as a semiotic sign is not a new concept, but it is an important one for this article. Indeed, for quite some time, researchers have looked at notions of modality, specifically the ways that different modes afford different potentials for meaning-making (Eisner, 1998; Jewitt & Kress, 2003). Embodiment is a mode that affords a multiplicity of meanings, including those that are simultaneously visual, kinesthetic, heard, sensed, felt, and lived. Additionally, embodied authorship is always multifaceted because there is always more than one mode involved in every form of information exchange; and because all authorship is influenced by the cultural, the social, the critical, and the historical (Barton et al., 2000; Kress, 2010; Street, 1995). So, though observers can interpret the embodied representations of a person's authorship, they can never fully translate it (Kress, 2010).

Moreover, Perry and Medina (2015) discuss in their book, how bodies simultaneously inscribe and are inscribed by social codes and cultural performances that get viewed by, shown to, remixed by, and re-contextualized by youth and children in particular moments in time. Drawing from the work of Gilles Deleuze and Felix Guattari (1987), Perry & Medina's work also suggests that bodies are constantly in motion (a state of becoming), relating to others. In other words, knowledge is not merely represented through bodies, knowledge is also created through embodiment. This bodied process is fundamental to meaning-making, but also to identity-making (Enriquez, Johnson, Kontovourki, & Mallozzi, 2016).

Barthes (1977) posited nearly 40 years ago that participants (in a situated context) not only interpret texts in relation to their own experiences, they also construct and add new information, transforming the original message, and thereby becoming authors. Authors, as he stated, are "both external and internal meaning-makers", including any person who contributes to the interpretation or actualization of a text, be it "declared, hidden, or withdrawn" (Barthes, 1977, p. 110). According to Barthes:

- Declared Participants: authors who are visibly creating meaning and contribute to the text within the social contexts. For example, the actors who act on the stage, or the child who writes a letter.
- Hidden Participants: the less visible authors who, though less obvious, play a part in shaping the text within the social contexts (Barthes, 1977). For example, the audience member who interprets the meaning of a play, claps at the end, and thereby influences the overall performance.
- Withdrawn Participants: authors who were once "dialogically" (Bakhtin, 1981) involved in contributing to the meaning-making. For example, the teacher who influenced the playwright and hence the creation of the play at an earlier time.

When thought about in this way, communication is continually being authored, and authorship is always embodied, semiotic, and relational – being both complexly received and remade at the same time.

Discursive embodied positions: bodies as situated and subjective

The cultural rituals of the context, the structured routines, as well as the space in which the practices take place all come into play when bodies inscribe and are inscribed by others. Authorship is dialogic (Bakhtin, 1981), socially situated, and subjective, influenced by the socio-critical experiences of the authors themselves, including their beliefs, histories, values, past conversations, actions, and interactions, as well as the contexts in which they communicate.

The children in the example above, not only come to know that "perfection is different for everybody" (every body), they also come to understand their own realities – that shops tend to have mannequins that are typically abled, lean, and attractive. At the same time, by comparing mannequins to the bodies of actual people, they begin to refute this socially constructed norm, thus forming their own opinions, re-actions, and ultimately their own identities.

The cultural rituals of the context, the structured routines, as well as the space in which the practices take place all come into play in an embodied discourse. Moreover, embodiment, where body image, affect, social relationships, and situated practices interplay always include power subjectivities, including the ways that people position each other and themselves.

When taking on various perspectives, people create storylines and imagine subject positions (Davies & Harré, 1990). These discursive embodied positions are not only dynamic and flexible in nature, they also have the potential to give authors a sense of belonging and a feeling of power. For example, an author might position himself/herself in one group and not in another (e.g. Leaders are important. I am a leader. Therefore, I am not a follower). Positioning the self and others gives the person the chance to include and exclude others and to feel the effects of these stances (e.g. She is a girl, not a boy. Therefore, she will align herself with this group of girls. Boys are not allowed here.) Discursive subject positions always occur in relation to a web of other influences, for example: (1) which modes are being explored; (2) who is involved; (3) what is the situated practice; and (4) how are others feeling.

Furthermore, identities are formed through discursive embodied positioning; the perspectives, actions, and emotions of the author combined with the ways that other people act/react or assume/assign subject positions all become part and parcel of the author's "figured world" (Holland, Lachicotte, Skinner, & Cain, 1998). Thus, identities then are bodily and multidimensional, layered constructed in dynamic ways and stemming from shifting circumstances. This is because discourse and affect are mutually consti-tuted in the production of knowing (Stein, 2008). In other words, the way an author feels about a particular topic will shape his or her embodied authorship, and ultimately reshape the entire experience as a whole, including his or her actions; the interactions of the participants; the constructed storylines created; the subject positions that are assigned and assumed (Winters & Vratulis, 2013).

Vignette #1: no ordinary loser!

Stories about body image were collected from several community organizations (e.g. a weight loss clinic, a yoga studio, a runner's group, a local college, a local university, a professional author/illustrator association). These stories took on many forms including films, photos, letters, narratives, and poems. They also covered a range of topics about body image – everything from big ears and wild hair to weight gain and hairy arms.

One study participant, a youth who was struggling with weight issues, submitted a transcript of a speech that she wrote for a school project. This speech entitled "No Ordinary Loser" made it to the annual regional speech competition. It placed 2nd overall. Melissa's speech spoke about how others called her overweight and made fun of her for being obese.

Below is a section of her speech.

> "Don't give up what you want the most for what you want in the moment." I say this quote to myself many times a day and over the past 5 months it has helped me tremendously. So what exactly do I want the "most?"

Well mid-August of the past year I made up my mind that what I really wanted the most was to be healthy. Many twelve year olds are not worrying about such a thing. They're too busy being active, being with friends and badgering their parents about getting the latest gadgets. This was not the case for me. My time and thoughts were consumed about feeling unwell. I had reached a very unhealthy weight. I was feeling angry and frustrated with myself. Although my parents and family are all very loving I was feeling very alone.

Good morning honourable judges, teachers, parents and students. Obesity is not a laughing matter. It destroys our health. Obesity can lead to high blood pressure, high cholesterol, diabetes, breathing problems and a whole lot more serious complications and illnesses. I knew that I was headed for many of these problems. Before the summer break last year, I noticed that I was having a hard time keeping up in gym class. I would get short of breath easily and I would be panting and taking rest periods when everyone else was still running around. I would use a puffer just so that I could be able to breathe normally. I knew this wasn't right but I didn't know how to fix it...I was also very involved in dance. However, I was never moved in up levels because I was told that I could not get my legs high enough or I wasn't flexible enough. I was laughed at because of the way I looked in my dance costumes and even when I wasn't at dance comments were made that I could not wear the latest fashions because they didn't come in my size. I would feel so upset about all this but the more upset I got the more I turned to food to help me through it....

Food comforted me but after eating the junk I felt even worse than I did before. It became a vicious circle. Then one day, in August I looked in the mirror, not just looked in the mirror but took a real hard look at myself. I don't know exactly what clicked but I made a promise to myself. I decided to make some changes.... I knew that I was a good person, inner beauty is what really matters and I'm a great kid but I had to make some changes to my outer self....

The narrative shown above was analyzed using a drama structure called Alter Ego, where three voices are portrayed simultaneously, including the protagonist herself (centre column), the negative thoughts expressed and in her head (left column), the positive thoughts expressed and in her head (right column). Analyzing the data through drama structures, as seen in Table 1, does a few things. First, it helps us (the authors) visualize the bodies of the participants, imaging how the dramatic scenes might physically be embodied and played out. Second, it provides a dialogic analytical approach that links to the theoretical elements of this paper – perceptions of body image, feelings, social actions, of subjective positions of the participants. Third, the voices themselves

Table 1. Case illustration analysis using alter-ego for "No Ordinary Loser".

Inner thought #1	Protagonist data	Inner thought #2
I was finding comfort in eating all those things that made me even heavier like chips, ice cream, and my favorite chocolate.	"Don't give up what you want the most for what you want in the moment?	Nothing tastes as good as being healthy.
I am not flexible enough. I am being laughed at because of how I look.	...I was never moved in up levels because I was told that I could not get my legs high enough.	I am a great kid, but I have to make some changes to my outer self.
Those thin-girl fashions do not come in my size.	...I could not wear the latest fashions."	Inner beauty is what really matters.
I come from two European backgrounds, where food is at the centre of everything.	"I was not sure how mom was going to react to my decision.	I was feeling overwhelmed by how much weight I would have to lose. But I was ready to change.
I would be panting and taking rest periods when everyone else was still running around. I would use a puffer just so that I could be able to breathe normally.	...Be the best you can be!"	My goal is not to look like a supermodel or an actress that has been air brushed in a magazine. I just want to be me, happy, healthy and an inspiration to as many young people who are going through the same thing I'm dealing with.

provide a commentary of the character's inner feelings and inner speech (cf. Neelands & Goode, 2000).

Above, Melissa, the declared author, created and performed a speech that expressed her challenges with weight loss. Hidden and withdrawn authors who participated in the dialogic conversation included Melissa's classmates who were the bullies and the witnesses of the bullying, her dance teacher, her family and her mother specifically, and even the weight loss group that helped shape her experiences.

The analysis demonstrates that Melissa's perceptions of body image and her bodily practices play a significant role in her daily life in- and out-side of the classroom. So much so, in fact that she decided to choose weight loss as her topic of discussion for her schooled speech event.

Speeches, by nature, are embodied. They are typically performed in front of an audience who not only listens, but also watches. Audiences witness the body postures, gestures, gazes, and facial expressions of the presenter – the performance itself. By performing a speech as a method of expression, Melissa contrasts the negative perceptions she feels/others feel about her image with the positive actions she has made in her life; at the same time, she compares her body with others. She demonstrates confidence and courage by putting herself in front of others and refusing to be discursively positioned in defeated or pitiful ways. Here, using her words and embodiment, Melissa re-positions herself as a survivor. Edmonstone (2016) examines the multifaceted ways we behave in order to avoid the emotional challenges of living with uncertainty. It is suggested in this research that learning arises from working at the edges between knowing (positive capability/performativity) and not-knowing (negative capability/performativity) because it offers the possibility of exposure to truth "in the moment" or insight. "It involves living with uncertainty, yet still ultimately acting in the world" (p. 139). In this way Melissa's speech is considered as an action-learning framework, which temporarily addresses her feelings of uncertainty, while at the same time, involves her in a relational conversation about body image with her peers and also positions her as someone who is able to refute the subjective perceptions of others.

Jones (2016) agrees that in any given situation, learning is constituted through an entanglement of bodies, space, emotions, material resources, and discursive subject stances. These assemblages shape social contexts, identities, actions, and even culture. Realities are bodied through enacted performances that can be heard, but also seen and felt, and integrated back into and through the bodies of others as well. Bodied performances affect others and hold emotional resonance. In this way, feelings are fluid, triggered and represented through one's own bodily responses and by witnessing the actions/re-actions of others. "Affective energy might manifest in the sheer joy that exudes from our bodies through uncontrollable laughter….it might also manifest as pain and anger through sobbing…either way, affective energy can be seen…reverberating and pulsing through our bodies and embedded within our bodies as part of the ways we 'come to know' and 'come to be' in the world" (Thiel, 2016, p. 94).

Melissa's speech does not exist as an endpoint; because each time it is performed it is "re-viewed" by her and others. In other words, the speech performance shows the body in an active web of doings: desiring, affecting, feeling, comparing, and relating to others. Furthermore, each time the speech is performed (re-lived) it imposes a profound change in the presenter herself and her audience, causing its intended meaning to reverberate outwardly, and perhaps even initiate more vibrations to be felt (Deleuze & Guattari, 1987).

Melissa speaks about being positioned by others as a victim in the beginning; according to her, she is called names and is made to feel belittled because of her weight. However, throughout the performance of the speech, her emotion builds, demonstrating that she is (in her own words) "No ordinary loser". Her words and emotions transform her; improved confidence is exemplified in the postures and gestures she presents. She illustrates, but also takes ownership of the situation, authoring to her audience through body language and speech that she always was and still is beautiful.

Vignette #2: conditional voices

Post-secondary students transformed community stories about body image (such as Melissa's speech) into a 45-minute play, which was then presented to elementary students (Grades 4–7). This devised theatre process took place weekly for three hours per week over 10 weeks. It is important to note that a devised play is a collective and unfolding process, meaning it is collaboratively designed, negotiated, produced, and disseminated. So, unlike more traditional forms of the theatre where a script originates from one writer and then is performed by a group, here the group of post-secondary students improvised and authored scenes that became more solidified and scripted. As this process "came to be", these declared authors positioned each other in social, affective, and critical ways.

Several scenes in the play offered alternative forms of expression of these bodily conditions through gestures/movement, scripted scene work, dance routines, monologues, and images. During two scenes in the play – the non-verbal scenes – the actors danced their understandings of bodily conditions such as amblyopia (lazy eye), leukemia, dyslexia, and hyperhidrosis (excessive sweating). These scenes illustrated both frustration and catharsis in relation to these conditions and included both the ways that the participants felt during their own past encounters and also the ways that others framed and spoke about their bodies. These dance scenes themselves were at times impulsive and sporadic, including sudden and angled movements, and also at other times sustained and flowing, including continuous and curved movements.

The participants, during the focus groups and interviews that followed, referred to their choreographed scenes as mirrored reflections, showing dichotomies such as the participants' inner feelings versus the reactions of others, and perceived negative and positive emotions. Drawing from this observation of the data, the following narrative case illustration uses a drama strategy called mirrors, which focuses on actions and their mirrored reflections (cf. Neelands & Goode, 2000). As seen below in Table 2, photographs and still shots from videos were placed side by side with the recorded interviews of the participants. Analyses focused on the participants' body image perceptions, affect, as well as the social and critical positions they assumed and assigned. More specifically, we highlighted the feelings that the participants in the dance/movement scenes used to describe their work, and then look carefully at chosen photos that captured these emotions.

The first part of the vignette represented a scene about having leukemia, including the emotions of courage and defeat. During the focus groups, the participants discussed

Table 2. Case illustration analysis using mirrors for "Conditional Voices".

Voiced to others (what is portrayed)	Image	Voiced to Self (what is spoken of outside the play)
"There's lots of pressure to look good. Some days I can handle that pressure." COURAGE	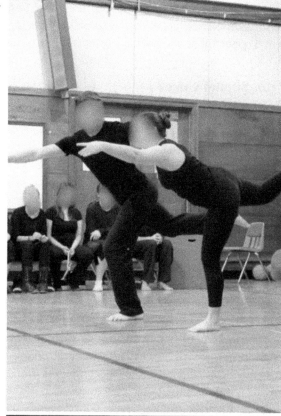	"Having no hair painted a target on me!" DEFEAT
"Kids need to feel confident in their own skin." SELF-ASSURANCE	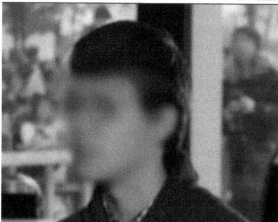	"At times it <u>was hard to</u> <u>feel</u> <u>confident.</u> <u>I grew up with</u> <u>an eye</u> <u>condition.</u>" FRUSTRATION

(*Continued*)

Table2. (Continued).

Voiced to others (what is portrayed)	Image	Voiced to Self (what is spoken of outside the play)
"Having sweaty hands is certainly not as serious or debilitating as traditionally recognized exceptionalities, so in many respects I am fortunate." HOPE	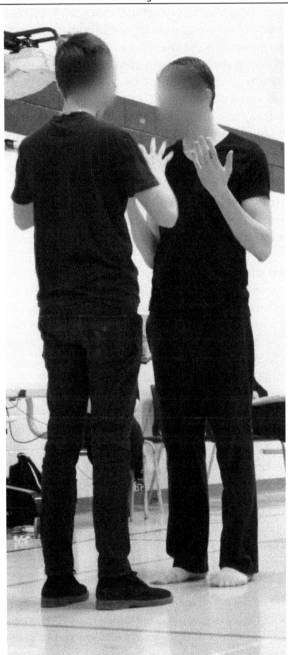	"Virtually everything I touch gets sweaty and yucky, and I cannot help it at all." HELPLESSNESS

ideas around what is a normal body versus an abnormal body. Additionally, they talked about peer pressure and being targeted when a body is perceived as "imperfect". Their movement work in the play and then their discussions that followed suggest that bodies are both representational and knowing – both "being" and "becoming" (Deleuze & Guattari, 1987). Perry and Medina (2015), extend this idea in their work. Drawing on performative pedagogies and sociocultural practices, they suggest that though bodies are often theorized in ways that stem from dualisms, they conceive bodies as whole, but also intricately relational to the world they inhabit.

The second scene in the vignette above demonstrates this idea. In an interview following a rehearsal, Sam (a post-secondary student) simultaneously discusses feelings of self-assurance and frustration based on his own perceptions of body image. While trying to convey a message of "kids needing to feel confident in their own skin", he struggles with his own physical challenges, having a condition called amblyopia. His input into the dancer's scene and his performance in the movement scene, aim to position the audience as "a confident and perfectly knowledgeable body of meaning-makers", and at the same time as outsiders who could never know his personal experiences with an "imperfect body" (a lazy eye). This dichotomy that he speaks about concurrently evokes feelings of both self-assuredness and security as well as frustration and insecurity – a mirrored relational affect, so to speak.

This mirrored affect is again physicalized in the third part of the vignette, where the condition of hyperhidrosis is also explored. Here the dancers in play are drawn together and then pulled apart, seamlessly so that the audience is not able to tell who is leading the actions and who is following. The intermingling bodies evoke feelings of hope and helplessness. The authorship is relational, as each person involved, including the participants, seem to animate each other.

These mirrored scenes invite broader notions of authorship as the dancers, alongside the audience members, influence the scenes and ultimately shape the play itself. The dancers, when asked later talked about how each audience was so different and how these audiences' reactions actually informed the energy that the dancers were feeling, and as a result shaped the piece itself. Thus, the audience (the more hidden authors) while actively interpreting the bodies on stage and reacting to the dancers' scene also had opportunities to expand, participate in, and even shape the piece itself. Here, bodily stories from the community became embodied narratives. Furthermore, these embodied stories when witnessed by an audience, became a part of a bigger cultural story about how bodies are rejected, accepted, shamed, and celebrated within school settings.

And all the while, the scenes themselves evoke emotions (as all art should) for both the actors and the audience about what it is like to live with conditions like leukemia, amblyopia (a lazy eye), and hyperhidrosis (excessive sweating) – conditions that make a person feel "imperfect". Here bodies are more than social texts that represent and are represented. For ideologies of body image also come into play – perceptions of what it is like to be imperfect and to compare oneself to an ideal. Indeed, bodies affect others and leave emotional residues. In this way, bodies are affective and relational; reminding us that embodiment is influenced by both the relationship in and between one's body, as well as its social context (Piran & Teall, 2012).

Vignette #3: let's just make them normal

In the third phase of the study, drama-in-education workshops were offered to elementary students in the region. These 55-minute workshops were specifically focused on a dramatic inquiry approach to learning called Mantle of the Expert (Heathcote & Bolton, 1995). Eight elementary schools were visited in total. The students ranged from Grades 4–7. During a mantle, a fictional world is created. Participants in the drama are asked to take on the role of experts in a designated field. Student authors in this study were asked to become expert designers: their goal, to design the perfect mannequin. In order to help them do this, at one point in the drama they were given templates to fill out together (Figure 1).

While sharing their templates, a student made a comment that upset and challenged others in the group. "We decided to make our mannequin a normal skin colour." Using a drama technique called hot seating, where a character is questioned about his behaviors and motivations, I transcribe the scene below in Table 3, and describe the event.

Bodies are storied within social contexts as people assume and assign subject positions (Davies & Harré, 1990). Over time, these positions become believed (and solidified) to some extent, forming identities. In this way, we acknowledge that identity is not something innate or uncovered, but rather an interactive and continually re-constructed process. This idea is highlighted by Holland et al. (1998); these authors suggest that identity is not housed inside of people, but rather that identity is continually re-constructed (or in their words – re-authored). They write:

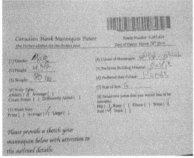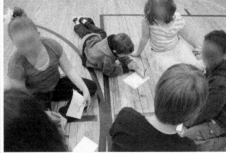

Figure 1. Imperfect/I'm perfect template.

Table 3. Case illustration analysis using hot seating for "Let's Just Make Them Normal".

Panel (audience)	Character (expert Mannequin designer)
What color should we make the mannequin?	
	Let's just make them normal.
Normal?	
	Yes. Normal color.
What's that supposed to mean?	
	Normal color, like skin color. Whitish-peach, you know!
Hey! I am not whitish-peach. And I seem normal.	
	Um...
You're being racist.	
	No. I'm not...I just meant...um...that's the color mannequins usually are...I mean in stores.

> The meaning that we make of ourselves is, in Bakhtin's terms, "authoring the self," and the site at which this authoring occurs is a space defined by the interrelationship of differentiated "vocal" perspectives on the social world (p. 173).

Here, drawing on Bakhtin (1981), these authors argue that identity is always dialogic – relational, multiple, and ongoing – and that within sociocultural environments identities are re-made.

The child in the vignette refers to the whitish-peach skin tone as "normal", which upsets others. Though the child goes on to explain himself, the others feel slighted by his insensitivity, and even position him as a racist. These emotions and subjective positions all play into how meaning is negotiated within that situated context.

Emotions of the participants became heated at times during the drama workshop. These situations were not handled as problems, but rather as opportunities for opening up critical and frank discussions about body image and bodies in schooled settings. Thinking critically about possible discursive positions not only has the potential to extend learning – as people encounter different points of view, but it also encourages empathy building. Here, students involved in the social context have opportunities to look both inside themselves (individual thoughts) and outside themselves (social relations) at the same time.

Discussion

In regard to the topic of body image and embodiment, this study uses drama and playbuilding to unpack how children and youth perceive their bodies within school contexts. Findings suggest that body image itself (i.e. how children perceive their bodies) and embodiment (i.e. how children use their bodies for communication and learning) are vital but often-invisible topics in schooled settings, where bodies are constructed, shamed, adored, and marginalized. Ninety-three percent of the study participants demonstrated through playbuilding, drama, discussion, and other art-based activities that they had negative thoughts about their bodies, and that these thoughts sometimes hampered the ways they interacted in schools. Emotions were evoked throughout the study as people affected others around them and felt the effects of bodies as well. Bodies were inscribing and inscribed upon at every turn. This embodied authorship helped to shape how the students (both post-secondary and elementary) narrated their own identities, as well as how their assumed and assigned discursive positions within the situated contexts.

Bodies are implicated in every subject in school. For example, in the introduction, Sofie, the girl with the cleft palette scar rarely lowered her hand. Others read this gesture and positioned her as shy and even too scared to participate. Yet, this is not the embodiment that the authors of this paper witnessed. In the first vignette that followed, Melissa faced challenges socially in regard to the weight she was carrying. Internally, it also affected her outlook on life and her schoolwork, and her identity. Yet, she rejected the perceptions that others had of her, and spoke back to them, both with actions and words. A section of the second vignette shows that Arron (a post-secondary student), when completing his schoolwork, often thought about a condition that he has, hyperhidrosis. During a follow-up interview, he spoke about how his sweaty palms made him feel nervous and inhibited. He did not want to pass a prop in drama class, handle a beaker in science class, or record notes in language arts class. He especially struggled in group projects, mentioning that he always kept his hands in his pockets; others perceived this body language as defiance and often positioned him as distant. Moreover, the third vignette demonstrates that even young children (8 year olds) are aware of their body image and the ways their bodies interact with others in social situations. Beliefs about their bodies, and hence their identities, were relational in the ways these children and behaved in schooled settings. Their beliefs and perceptions influenced their thoughts and feelings, their behaviours and actions, and hence, their discussions, and the texts that they create.

Post-secondary and elementary students consistently and fluidly make observations regarding bodies/body images, including how they feel about their own bodies. These observations are dependent on perceptions that have been formed by the media, by their personal histories and cultures, and by the situated contexts at hand. Even in school settings, their perceptions often foreground the bodily, social, affective, and critical ways that study participants story their identities about their bodies.

Children and youth use their bodies to represent their thoughts and feelings, but also to understand and support one another (e.g. through proximity or body positions) and to communicate too (relate to, react to, align with, sense, reject). Moreover, children consistently positioned themselves and others invoking actions and evoking emotional reactions.

How, then, might educators teach children in authentic ways that consider students' perceptions of their bodies as well as their bodily ways of knowing, and at the same time allow students to communicate and express their inner thoughts in schools? Perhaps one solution includes paying attention to bodies, and paying attention to embodied ways of knowing. Drama and the arts offer unique opportunities to express beliefs, ideas, and feelings through embodiment (Lenters & Winters, 2013; Medina & Campano, 2006).

However, as this study shows, drama is not perfect and can hold a host of challenges too. For example, drama has the potential to plunk people into situations that are outside their comfort zones. Sam, for example, in the second vignette, wanted to narrate his feelings about his lazy eye to the audience, whereby at the same time, he was aware that these children would be looking at his eye and even judging him. Drama puts bodies at the forefront; this can be problematic when there is a lot of pressure to look good in today's media-driven society. Though drama offers unique opportunities for learning about others and chances to be feel human, it also has the potential to put a target on people because it asks them to take risks and share opinions on difficult subjects. Arron acknowledged that drama provided him a way to share his fears and build understanding about his medical condition, and at the same time, it embarrassed him. "Virtually everything I touch gets sweaty and then people think I am gross."

Drama activities can also offer perspectives that might lead to uncomfortable situations. In the third vignette, Franky had to defend his opinions about skin tones and mannequin design. Indeed, by using drama in this study, we observed his perceptions about mannequins. And as a result we witnessed children getting emotionally invested, negotiating within situated contexts, positioning themselves and others, and demonstrating/discussing affect. At the same time, the majority of study participants we interviewed (both youth and children), felt that although drama held its own challenges, it was worth exploring as safe artful practices provided opportunities for differentiated instruction, creativity, and access to critical engagement and authentic expression.

This study demonstrates that child participants whose bodies were abled, fairer, and physically athletic were positioned as "more popular" and "closer to perfect" by their peers. Without a doubt, this study demonstrates that individuals and groups have pre-conceived perceptions of how bodies should move and be thought about.

Finally, this study suggests that notions of bodies and embodiment, in schools, are in urgent need of theorizing – especially in ways that are intrinsically linked to the perceived, affective, relational, and critical ways that people represent meanings and come to know their worlds. Embodied practices in school settings need to be looked at as complexly intertwined, providing potentials for social, critical, emotionally responsive, learning opportunities.

In an attempt to touch upon the lived, affective, and tacit nature of embodiment, this study also uses dramatic structures of analysis. These structures do, to some extent, what drama does – they provide opportunities to see multiple perspectives simultaneously, and to understand the discursive positions of participants. Though these methods of analyses could use some refining, they invite conversations about bodies and embodied research.

Conclusion

This article explores not only how dramatic approaches to communication and learning influence the perceived, affective, social, and critical assemblages that children and youth construct, shaping their identities and informing their schooled practices, but also how these creative forms are communicated, designed, negotiated, shared, cen-sored, and refuted in various school communities (i.e. post-secondary and elementary schools). Findings demonstrate three main points. First, bodies are implicated in all areas of education. Many educators take for granted that students are comfortable with their bodies in schools, yet this study demonstrates that high numbers of students are not comfortable with the ways they look or how their body is perceived by their peers when they are interacting in schools. How will students perform an activity when there is some aspect that they do not like about their body? Is it fair that insecure students be held to the same performance standards as their more confident peers? Educators need to remember that though not acknowledged, the body, emotions, and socio-critical posi-tions of power and vulnerability are omnipresent and are in every classroom conversa-tion or lesson. Some students struggle with their bodies, and thus will struggle with their expression when communicating and performing schooled tasks.

Second, the Arts offer educators and scholars ways to challenge firmly held and narrowly defined definitions of authorship. Specifically, drama and playbuilding (and other creative forms) encourage broader ideals about bodily perceptions, affect, social collaborations, and power relations. The study clearly demonstrates that drama is not perfect either. On the one hand, drama has the potential to provide a stage for exploring participatory relationships, agency, and critical insights in classrooms, but on the other hand it also has the potential to shut down communication, initiating participants' feelings of fear and vulnerability, as well as sometimes encourage power inequities.

A third finding is that making sense of the complexities of children's and young adults' meaning-making is challenging. Embodied pedagogies such as playbuilding and drama suggest that bodies act on the world, but are also acted upon. Here, the concept of learning is inseparable from corporeal, emotionally resonant, cultural, and critical practice. The fields of embodiment and embodied authorship are in need of further theorizing to include fuller understandings of reality, including bodily ways of communicating and feeling within participatory and situated settings that are embedded in relations of power, history, and culture.

The smaller study contributes to the larger, international CAZ study by demonstrating that theories of embodiment have the potential to inform notions of authorship in schooled communities, and further, illustrating that all authorship is multimodal, lived (or improvised), and participatory. Additionally, this study suggests that when embodied pedagogies are used within communities, the arts and literacy are not as separate as school systems sometimes make them out to be. The arts and literacy both have the potential to connect broader notions of authorship, creativity, embodiment, affect, critical thinking, and situated community practice. And both require sensitivity and thought so that students can feel safe when they are asked to present, report, move, and perform in front of others.

Disclosure statement

No potential conflict of interest was reported by the authors.

Funding

This work was supported by the Social Sciences and Humanities Research Council of Canada [grant number 430-2013-1025].

References

Ahmed, S. (2004). Foreword. In M. Perry & C. L. Medina (Eds.), *Methodologies of Embodiment* (pp. xiii–xvi). New York, NY: Routledge.

Bakhtin, M. (1981). *The dialogic imagination: Four essays*. Austin, TX: University of Texas Press.

Barthes, R. (1977). *Image, music, text*. London: Fontana.

Barton, D., Hamilton, M., & Ivanic, R. (2000). *Situated literacies: Reading and writing in context*. London: Routledge.

Cash, T. F., & Pruzinsky, T. (2002). *Body image: A handbook of theory, research, and clinical practice.* New York, NY: Guilford Press, c2002.

Davies, B., & Harré, R. (1990). Positioning: The discursive production of selves. *Journal for the Theory of Social Behaviour, 20*(1), 43–63. doi:10.1111/jtsb.1990.20.issue-1

Deleuze, G., & Guattari, F. (1987). Devising in the Rhizome. In M. Perry & C. L. Medina (Eds.), *Methodologies of embodiment* (pp. 14–27). New York, NY: Routledge.

Edmonstone, J. (2016). Action learning, performativity and negative capability. Action Learning: Research and Practice, 13(2), 139–147.

Eisner, E. (1998). *The kind of schools we need: Personal essays.* Portsmouth, NH: Heinemann.

Enriquez, G., Johnson, E., Kontovourki, S., & Mallozzi, C. A. (Eds.). (2016). *Literacies, learning, and the body: Putting theory and research into pedagogical practice.* New York, NY: Routledge.

Gallagher, K. (2015). Foreword. In M. Perry & C. L. Medina (Eds.), *Methodologies of embodiment* (pp. xiii–xvi). New York, NY: Routledge.

Grushka, K. (2011). The "Other" literacy narrative: The body and the role of image production. *English Teaching Practice and Critique, 10*(3), 113–128.

Heathcote, D., & Bolton, G. (1995). *Drama for learning: Dorothy Heathcote's Mantle of the Expert approach to education.* Portsmouth, NH: Heinemann.

Hochchild, A. (1983). Foreword. In M. Perry & C. L. Medina (Eds.), *Methodologies of embodiment* (pp. xiii–xvi). New York, NY: Routledge.

Holland, D., Lachicotte, J., Skinner, D., & Cain, C. (1998). *Identity and agency in cultural worlds.* Cambridge: Harvard University Press.

Jacobson, H. L., Hall, M. L., Anderson, T. L., & Willingham, M. M. (2016). Religious beliefs and experiences of the body: An extension of the developmental theory of embodiment. *Mental Health, Religion & Culture, 19*(1), 52–67. doi:10.1080/13674676.2015.1115473

Jewitt, C., & Kress, G. (Eds.). (2003). *Multimodal literacy* (Vol. 4). New York, NY: Peter Lang.

Jones, S. (2016). When the body acquires pedagogy and it hurts: Discursive practices and material effects of round robin reading. In G. Enriquez, E. Johnson, S. Kontovourki, & C. A. Mallozzi (Eds.), *Literacies, learning, and the body: Putting theory and research into pedagogical practice.* New York, NY: Routledge.

Kress, G. (2010). *Multimodality.* London: Routledge.

Lenters, K., & Winters, K. L. (2013). Fracturing writing spaces: Multimodal storytelling ignites process writing. *The Reading Teacher, 67*(3), 227–237. doi:10.1002/TRTR.1210

Liechty, J. M., & Lee, M. (2013). Longitudinal predictors of dieting and disordered eating among young adults in the *U.S. International Journal of Eating Disorders, 46*(8), 790–800. doi:10.1002/eat.22174

Medina, C., & Campano, G. (2006). Performing identities through drama and teatro practices in multilingual classrooms. *Language Arts, 83*(4), 332–341.

Murnen, S. K., Smolak, L., Mills, J. A., & Good, L. (2003). Thin, sexy women and strong, muscular men: Grade-school children's responses to objectified images of women and men. *Sex Roles, 49* (9/10), 427–437. doi:10.1023/A:1025868320206

Neelands, J., & Goode, T. (2000). *Structuring drama work.* Cambridge, UK: Cambridge University Press.

Pahl, K., & Rowsell, J. (2012). *Literacy and Education.* New York, NY: Sage.

Perry, M., & Medina, C. L. (2011). Embodiment and performance in pedagogy research: Investigating the possibility of the body in curriculum experience. *Journal of Curriculum Theorizing, 27*(3), 62–75.

Perry, M., & Medina, C. L. (2015). *Methodologies of embodiment: Inscribing bodies in qualitative research.* New York, NY: Routledge.

Piran, N., & Teall, T. (2012). The developmental theory of embodiment. In G. McVey, M. P. Levine, N. Piran, & H. B. Ferguson (Eds.), *preventing eating-related and weight-related disorders: Collaborative research, advocacy, and policy change* (pp. 246–291). Waterloo, ON: Wilfred Laurier Press.

Selfie. (2013). In English Oxford online dictionary. Retrieved from https://en.oxforddictionaries.com/definition/selfie

Siegel, M., Kontovourki, S., Schmier, S., & Enriquez, G. (2008). Literacy in motion: A case-study of a shape-shifting kindergartener. *Language Arts, 86*(2), 89–98.

Smolak, L., & Thompson, J. K. (2009). *Body image, eating disorders, and obesity in youth. [electronic resource]: Assessment, prevention, and treatment.* Washington, DC: American Psychological Association, c2009.

Smolak, L., Levine, M., & Thompson, J. (2001). The use of the sociocultural attitudes towards appearance questionnaire with middle school boys and girls. *International Journal of Eating Disorders, 29*(2), 216–223. doi:10.1002/1098-108X(200103)29:2<216::AID-EAT1011>3.0.CO;2-V

Stein, P. (2008). *Multimodal pedagogies in diverse classrooms: Representation, rights, and resources.* London: Routledge.

Street, B. (1995). *Social literacies.* London: Longman.

Thiel, J. (2016). Shrinking in, spilling out, and living through: Affective energy in multimodal literacies. In G. Enriquez, E. Johnson, S. Kontovourki, & C. A. Mallozzi (Eds.), *Literacies, learning, and the body: Putting theory and research into pedagogical practice.* New York, NY: Routledge.

Woodcock, C. (2010). "I Allow Myself to FEEL Now ...": Adolescent girls' negotiations of embodied knowing, the female body, and literacy. *Journal of Literacy Research, 42*(4), 349–384. doi:10.1080/1086296X.2010.524856

Winters, K. (2010). Quilts of authorship: A literature review of multimodal assemblage in the field of literacy education. *Canadian Journal for New Scholars in Education, 3*(1). Retrieved from http://www.cjnse-rcjce.ca/ojs2/index.php/cjnse/article/viewArticle/161

Winters, K., & Vratulis, V. (2013). "Puppets don't have legs! Dinosaurs have digits!" Using the dramatic and media arts to deepen knowledge in content areas. *Education Matters: The Journal of Teaching and Learning, 1*(2), 91–110.

Playlinks: a theatre-for-young audiences artist-in-the-classroom project

Debra McLauchlan[†]

ABSTRACT

Playlinks, the project documented in this paper, contributed a theatre-based artist-in-the-classroom study to the Community Arts Zone initiative. *Playlinks* involved 248 elementary school classrooms in pre- and post-production workshops connected to live theatre that visited their schools. Data sources included researcher field notes, teacher evaluation forms, and interviews with both teachers and theatre personnel. Findings focus on teacher perceptions of three topics: (a) student engagement, (b) learning across cognitive and affective domains, and (c) benefits for teachers. The discussion section addresses implementation problems related to artist-in-the-classroom projects.

Introduction

Why is it important that school children experience the arts beyond participating as audience members? According to Eisner (2005), the arts receive very little attention in schools (p. 77). I write this paper as both a university researcher and grandmother of two youngsters under the age of five. My grandchildren, as all young children, engage naturally in the arts – as performers. With neither provocation nor self-censure, they sing, dance, draw, and make music. They learn from role play about life's occupations and routine activities, like shopping and driving a car. They unconsciously value their active experience of the arts, and do not separate arts-based pursuits from regular daily tasks.

And yet my 30-year experience in classrooms, as both teacher and teacher educator, tells me that school will teach my grandchildren that the arts are not important areas of study. Many of their teachers, themselves unfamiliar with the arts, will focus on paper-and-pencil preparation for standardized high-stakes tests (Betts, 2005), and some will consider practices like drama an invitation for classroom chaos and student misbehaviour (McLauchlan, 2006, p. 133.). Greene (2011) has proposed that contemporary educational aims, focused on "the manageable, the predictable, and the measurable", create an atmosphere in schools that is incompatible with the experience of art (p. 34). Formal education will also enculturate my grandchildren to the belief that creating art is a pursuit reserved for a talented few, blessed with a gift that is impossible to teach or

---

[†]Deceased

learn. However, research tells us otherwise – in particular for the purpose of this paper, research related to theatre-for-young audiences (TYA). This paper contributes to investigations addressing teachers' and students' responses to TYA initiatives (e.g. Bedard, 2011; Brinda & Whordley, 2005; Harvey & Miles, 2009; Horitz, 2006; Jackson, 2011; Klein, 2011; McLauchlan, 2009; Omasta, 2009).

Background to the *Playlinks* project

Playlinks was an artist-in-the-classroom initiative that involved elementary students in pre- and post-production workshops designed to enhance their experience of theatre. The project comprised a partnership between Carousel Players (a TYA company) and 41 Southern Ontario elementary schools. Students from 248 classrooms experienced theatre in a three-stage sequence. Stage 1 was a pre-production workshop: a classroom visit from an actor who presented two activities related to a script's content and/or themes. Stage 2 was the play's performance, viewed by all classes at the same time. Stage 3 was the post-production workshop: a classroom visit from an actor who presented three drama-based activities designed to deepen students' understanding of the play.

Primarily a touring company for elementary schools in Southern Ontario, Carousel Players has for almost 50 years provided what is often the first theatre experience for children aged 4–14. Carousel Players began as a semi-professional troupe-based company, whose members, guided by local playwrights and an artistic director, collaboratively created up to six productions per year. Audience participation was a central feature of these early scripts; to prepare children for the performance, actors regularly visited classrooms before a school viewed the play en masse. To continue children's exploration of a play, actors often re-visited classrooms after a performance. Carousel Players' early mandate included "intimate participatory theatre, preparatory and follow-up activities, [and] plays for the company by the company ..." (Coopman, 1989, p. 9).

Carousel Players gradually evolved from a local troupe-based company to a fully professional organization. As such, its current directors, designers, and actors are almost always professional union members. At present, it tours two to four performances per school year, with actors cast through professional audition processes. Audience participation has lost its centrality in Carousel Players productions. Play development remains a focus of the company's mandate; however, scripts are currently crafted over 2–3 years, in collaborations involving professional playwrights, directors, actors, and designers hired at various stages of the creative process.

In 2013, artistic director Pablo Felices-Lunes decided to revive pre- and post-production classroom visits, primarily because of his desire to intensify children's experiences of theatre. He envisioned *Playlinks* as a program wherein actors would: (a) introduce central concepts of a play in pre-show visits to each classroom and (b) continue students' participation in the play through interactive post-production activities:

> I brought forward an artistic vision statement saying that we really want to focus on our audiences and make sure that everything we do has a filter of asking, 'What is our audience getting? ... Are we serving them or not?' So we looked at ways to deepen their experience and came up with Playlinks. The hope was that by increasing the time and depth of the experience that an audience has with theatre, there would be a greater investment in the experience. (Interview Transcript, 14 February 2014)

By funding actors to implement classroom workshops, the Ontario Trillium Foundation allowed *Playlinks* to launch in January 2014. I devised the workshops for each production and trained actors to implement them in elementary classrooms. A single actor conducted each workshop; however, five actors were hired to accommodate multiple school settings and actor availability across the project's 4-month span. Because the success of artist-led workshops often hinges on artists' teaching capabilities (Upitis & Smithram, 2003, p. 49), a selection criterion for artists was instructional experience with children.

Simultaneously to Carousel Players' *Playlinks* initiative, Brock University Professor Jennifer Rowsell designed a government-funded project named Community Arts Zone (CAZ), involving an international team of researchers to examine the efficacy of arts-based projects in enhancing student literacy. Becoming affiliated with CAZ broadened *Playlinks'* scholarly scope, inviting me to analyse its capacity to enrich audience experience in an academic fashion.

Methodology and data collection

Playlinks focused on the capacity of pre- and post-production artist-led workshops to enhance student involvement in theatre that they experienced as audience members. This study adopted a mixed-method design (Creswell, 2012, p. 534), including both quantitative and qualitative data. Four sources contributed data to the study: (a) my classroom observational field notes of 10 workshops, (b) quantitative scores from 248 teacher evaluation forms, (c) open-ended written comments from the same 248 teachers, and (d) semi-structured interviews with 16 teachers, 2 Carousel Players' staff members (artistic director and general manager), and 2 *Playlinks* artists.

For each of the two productions involved in the study, I recorded field notes of two workshops in each of five different schools. I visited schools that spanned a wide geographical and socio-economic range, and observed workshops in all grade levels. Teachers in all *Playlinks* classrooms completed an evaluation form following each post-show workshop. The form consisted of two parts: (a) a Likert-scale (Mertler & Charles, 2005, p. 156) rating of statements probing teachers' opinions of the workshops' age and grade appropriateness, links to literacy (as part of the CAZ mandate), and enhancement of students' experiences of the play; and (b) a space for written comments about the workshops. Following the workshops, I returned to 16 schools to interview teachers across grade levels on their perceptions of the workshops' effects. The presence of Likert-scale quantitative measures of success was included in the study in order to satisfy the expectations of the Ontario Trillium Foundation, which requested specific indicators of the project's success. I do not report on quantitative dimensions of the research in this article.

Researcher perspective

Researcher integrity entails acknowledging biases and assumptions (Bogdan & Biklen, 1998; Kvale & Brinkmann, 2009) in the planning, conducting, and reporting of research. To enhance transparency of my perspective as a researcher in the present study, I hereby reveal aspects of my personal and professional life.

The power of theatre to deeply touch young people resonates with my personal history. My childhood, characterized by poverty and alcoholism, would definitely be labelled underprivileged. However, blessed with a photographic memory and a penchant for language, I accelerated through elementary grades, all the while feeling little connection to my school surroundings. Secondary school held no relevance for me, and I became a persistent thorn in the side of my teachers, two of whom threatened me with expulsion if I didn't attend class more often. One evening, because no cost was involved, I attended a school field trip to a major theatrical production. Seated at the back of the auditorium, I purposely surrounded myself with classmates who could be counted on to misbehave. But then the lights went down, and an enormous curtain opened on a translucent scrim, and gradually emerged a purplish brush of sky, and a starkly peaked roof with a ragged fiddler perched on top. He began to play, and I lost my capacity to speak, to move, and at times, to breathe. Throughout the performance, I sat riveted and unaware of my surroundings. I said nothing on the way home, and didn't sleep that night, awake in the certain knowledge that I was going to be somehow involved in theatre for the rest of my life.

After attending university on a scholarship, I became a secondary school drama teacher. Fifteen years in secondary classrooms taught me the capacity of theatre to enhance student engagement and motivation to learn across academic and affective domains (McLauchlan, 2001). For a few years, I also spent time in elementary classrooms, demonstrating drama techniques to teachers who requested my presence. While there, I learned that students were hungry and eager to participate in activities that allowed them to explore and communicate ideas through an artistic medium.

Over time, I pursued graduate studies in drama/theatre education. When, 15 years ago, my local university initiated a tenure-track position in drama education, I dove into a professional journey that allows me to explore the pedagogical power of drama and theatre through the lens of rigorous academic protocol. An important aspect of my approach to scholarly rigor is the mitigation of researcher preconceptions through bias-free data collection techniques.

In the present study, I was careful to solicit both teacher questionnaire and interview responses through neutrally worded prompts (Kvale & Brinkmann, 2009; Neuman, 2007). In the analysis of data, I focused primary attention on teacher quotations to determine emergent finding categories.

Summary of pre- and post-production workshops

Playlinks performances included two scripts selected by the company's artistic director: *Dib and Dob and the Journey Home* (Craig & Morgan, 1998) for Junior/Kindergarten to Grade 3 (ages 4–8), and *The Power of Harriet T.* (Miller, 1993/2013) for Grades 4–8 (ages 8–14). Workshop material invited students to participate in activities that allowed them to imagine and embody circumstances related to the plays.

Pre-production workshops generally occurred 2–3 days before the play's performance; post-production workshops, 2–3 days afterwards. In some cases, schools combined classes to participate in the post-production workshops. Workshops were sometimes scheduled on days when regular teachers were attending professional development sessions outside the school, and classes were supervised by supply teachers.

Dib and Dob and the Journey Home tells the story of two brothers who speak a unique language and, lost in a forest, encounter problems in finding their way home. Pre-production activities introduced students to the idea that spoken language is communicated both visually and orally, through the body as well as the voice. Students were challenged to decipher gibberish by attending to facial expression, gesture, and tone of voice. Because the play includes a monster, and the target audience included young children, students also learned a "monster-repellent" chant to repeat silently during the play, in the event that a monster should frighten them. Post-production activities deepened the play's communication focus by inviting children to create and decipher visual emotional cues. In various sized groups, students then used their bodies to portray objects found in the play. Next, they generated live "photographs" of Dib and Dob's adventures, in correct sequence. They problem-solved to suggest reasons for events in the play and discussed the characters' sibling relationship.

The Power of Harriet T. portrays episodes in the life of Underground Railroad heroine, Harriet Tubman. Pre-production activities introduced the Underground Railroad, and invited students to embody physical positions of power and powerlessness. Post-production activities returned to the notion of power by (a) having groups prepare tableaux representing moments of power and powerlessness in the play and (b) engaging students in a "voices-in-the-head" (Neelands, 1990, p. 61) activity wherein they vocalized recalled dialogue that invoked feelings of either power or powerlessness. Students then created a chant with movement to describe Harriet's actions and personal qualities. The workshop ended by inviting students to write letters to Harriet Tubman.

Findings

Previous research has described the importance of teacher attitudes and perceptions in optimizing students' experience of the arts (Andrews, 2010; Betts, 2005; Saldaña, 1995). Focusing on teacher responses to the *Playlinks* workshops, findings emerged from four sources: observational field notes; teacher evaluation from quantitative scores; teacher evaluation from qualitative comments; and interview transcripts from 16 teachers, Carousel Players' artistic director and general manager, and two *Playlinks* artists. For the purposes of this article, I have not drawn on quantitative data.

Findings from all sources here are merged into three general categories of teacher opinion: (a) student engagement, (b) learning across cognitive and affective domains, and (c) benefits for teachers.

Student engagement

Engagement is "[t]he extent to which students actively and persistently participate in learning ..." (Walberg, 2011, p. 96). Signs of student engagement include "an absence of irrelevant behavior", "concentration on tasks", and "enthusiastic contributions" (p. 96). All data sources emphasized the capacity of artist-led activities to generate student engagement. Teachers first praised the pre-production workshops' effectiveness in creating excitement about the play that students were about to see:

[The pre-show workshop] made [the students] more excited. They wanted to know what was going to happen …. (Grade 1 teacher)

Post-performance workshops were both active and interactive. My field notes documented that most students seemed highly involved in the activities. The workshops' active component elevated students' participation from audience members to "vocally, verbally, and physically" (McCaslin, 2006, p. 10) engaged arts-makers. Embodied involvement sparked essential qualities of what Bundy (2003) labelled "aesthetic engagement": "connection, animation, and heightened awareness" (p. 180). Connection arose when students "experience[d] and read the events of drama against their own prior life experiences and understandings" (p. 180). Animation promoted "a feeling of invigoration" evident in facial expression and body language (p. 180). Heightened awareness manifested as an openness to explore aspects of humanity that had not previously been considered (p. 180).

An apparent cause of engagement was the workshops' requirement for students to work co-operatively in various peer groupings. The collaborative creation of aesthetic responses to artists' prompts appeared to be an unusual and welcomed opportunity. Teachers not only praised the artists' ability to encourage peer interaction in the workshops but also related collaborative participation to their engagement in the activities:

The students were engaged & got to participate actively together in 'acting' out. (Grade 1/2 teacher)
The students were very engaged and interested in the workshop [because it was] very interactive! (Grade 6 teacher)

Learning across cognitive and affective domains

Artist-implemented activities engage students in experiences that may enhance learning across wide-ranging objectives (Lushington, 2003; Rabkin & Redmond, 2006; Upitis & Smithram, 2003). "The arts are cognitive activities, guided by human intelligence, that make unique forms of meaning possible" (Elsner, 2005, p. 75). All *Playlinks* data sources concurred that workshops facilitated learning. In the cognitive domain, teachers especially valued the reinforcement of curriculum content:

When the children were working on their tableaux, they were focusing on the concept of beginning, middle, and end. And that connected very well with our [language arts] curriculum. (Grade 2 teacher)
There were curriculum links to drama, dance, oral expression or oral language. There were links to music. There were links to literacy. There were links to social studies. [The workshops] were the perfect kind of activity because they included a lot of curriculum expectations in one session. (Grade 6 teacher)

Post-production workshops encouraged students to recall and ask questions about important aspects of the plays:

[The workshop] gave [students] a chance to talk about the play with their classmates and demonstrate their thinking about how they perceived … events that were portrayed. (Grade 5 teacher)
[Students] had an opportunity to ask questions and revisit really important scenes in the play. (Grade 3 teacher)

Much *Playlinks* activity investigated social issues embedded in the two plays. Workshop material for *Dib and Dob and the Journey Home* explored both interpersonal communication and sibling relationships. *The Power of Harriet T.* workshops focused on power imbalance and the development of inner personal strength. Teachers praised the issue-based aspect of *Playlinks*, especially when the issues supported curricular objectives:

> We looked for clues in facial expressions & body language to tell how we know how people were feeling. Inferring and finding clues has been a focus in our literacy activities. (Grade 2 teacher)
> The workshop fits nicely into social issues covered in Grade 7/8. (Grade 7/8 teacher)

Of particular power was the students' physical embodiment of issues related to the plays:

> The tableau exercise helped [students] to communicate through body language. I think it helped them to understand that place where we have all been when we feel that we are not appreciated, that we are denigrated or under someone's foot. (Grade 6 teacher)

Fostered by opportunities to communicate aesthetically through structured, colla-borative, and embodied activities, students became affectively engaged in the work-shops. Affective engagement "reaches the emotional and belief system aspects of those who facilitate and participate in it" (Tooman, 2010, para. 2), thus promoting an exam-ination of "attitudes, appreciations, values, and emotional sets or biases" (Krathwohl, Bloom, & Masia, 1964, p. 7).

> The workshops tapped into character education, and trying to understand others and develop empathy. ... Respecting people and understanding our responsibility to treat everyone with fairness and equity. (Grade 7 teacher)
> [The workshops] hit a lot of expectations as far as personal and social skills and awareness of emotions. (Grade 3 teacher)

Issue-based activities made theatre more meaningful to students by inviting them to relate ideas to their own experiences:

> [The post-show workshop] made connections for the class. For example, the connection between feeling emotions and how we show those emotions [through gesture and tone of voice]. (Grade 1 teacher)
> My colleague and I were talking about the [activity] when the students had to speak as a voice in Harriet's head .... And at first there was a whole string of [negative] statements, 'I'm not worth anything', 'I stink', 'I suck', and those seemed to come quite freely. And then as it progressed, there were stronger voices, saying positive things, like 'I can do anything I want to', 'If only I dream, I believe', that sort of thing. And that picked up pace and it was really beautiful to hear that sort of transition in [students'] thinking and feeling. (Grade 6 teacher)

Benefits for teachers

Although *Playlinks'* major intention was to enhance student's experience of live theatre, findings reveal that teachers benefitted from the experience as well. First, they perceived artist-led workshops as a form of professional development, primarily because drama is a required component of the Ontario curriculum that most teachers feel insufficiently prepared to teach (Campbell & Townshend, 1997; McLauchlan, 2009; Patteson, 2005).

I'm not comfortable [teaching] drama. It was nice to see how the artist presented information and now I can copy the activities myself. (Grade 7/8 teacher)

We're not experts in drama. [The artist] gave us ideas and added to our [instructional] repertoire. (Grade 5 teacher)

Secondly, teachers learned about their students by observing responses to someone in authority other than themselves:

It's good when you can observe your students without having to be in charge. I was able to see students in a way that I don't normally get to see them. (Grade 3 teacher)

Thirdly, teachers appreciated the workshops' reinforcement of curriculum content, particularly in language arts, social studies, drama, and character education:

For my grade level, with regard to literacy, the workshop worked very well. There were links to media literacy, critical understanding of points of view, drama, and oral communication. (Grade 6 teacher)

Finally, two teachers commented on the effectiveness of the workshops in providing drama assessment for their students' report cards:

I can use what I saw the students doing as part of their drama mark. I can use the workshops as part of their evaluation.

Discussion

Based on teacher response data, *Playlinks* appears to have successfully met its goals of enriching and deepening students' experiences of theatre. This section of the paper focuses on two aspects of the project: (a) factors related to student learning through drama-based activities and (b) optimal conditions for conducting artist-in-the-classroom initiatives.

According to Omasta (2009), professional TYA companies have a responsibility "… to serve as pedagogues, teaching children about theatre and aesthetics, contributing to their social development in a diverse world, and incorporating links to school curricula" (pp. 113–114.) Teachers' responses to *Playlinks* workshops support claims of the benefits of theatre to enhance student learning across the curriculum.

"[D]rama is a way of knowing – and often a more stimulating way than that offered through the distanced, abstract learning provided in a purely intellectual approach" (Brockett, 1985, p. 3). Inviting students to enter actively and imaginatively into the lives of others promotes "a more intense learning experience, because it calls on [a mixture of] emotional, imaginative, and intellectual capacities and thereby impresses itself more firmly on [the] senses … (p. 3). Learning through drama does not spring from a singularly intellectual source, but rather evolves "during a comprehensive process that entails the whole body/mind" (Tuisku, 2015, p. 16). Moreover, entering drama does not entail "an 'intention to learn'. It is an intention to create or take part in or solve something" (Bolton, 1984, p. 154).

Thus, drama offers a unique "space for enquiry" (Cahill, 2014, p. 35) that defies the separation of curriculum into distinct subject areas. Rather, drama facilitates "deep learning" across subjects, because it invites students to "blend" their own life understandings with those of dramatized characters (Duffy, 2014, p. 98). "… [L]earning through drama gives students a lived, co-created physically engaging, imaginatively alive, and personally relevant experience onto which students can map the curriculum" (p. 97).

However, "[i]t is difficult to determine drama-centered instruction's impact on student learning with absolute certainty … (Duffy, 2014, p. 97). Insights gained through drama activities may "bring about shifts in perspective and … sow seeds for the making of meaning which won't necessarily germinate at the site of the experience but may grow and bear much fruit later" (Cusworth & Simons, 1997, p. 68). *Playlinks* teachers appeared to appreciate the intrinsic value of the workshops as much as the curriculum connections they made.

Artist-in-the-classroom projects that are tied to theatrical productions, such as *Playlinks*, may be considered Theatre In Education (TIE), a movement that began in Britain in the mid-1960s (Jackson, 2005). The major aim of TIE is "to provide an experience for children that will be intensely absorbing, challenging, even provocative, and an unrivalled stimulus for further work on the chosen subject in and out of school" (Jackson, 2005, p. 1). In North America, one successful example of a sustained TIE program is The Creative Arts Team, an educational theatre company that "aims to motivate urban youth to examine pertinent curricular themes and social issues" through participatory drama workshops connected to theatrical performances (Riherd & Hardwick, 2005, p. 205). Other TIE projects have been documented in Canada (Fairhead, 2005), Australia (O'Toole & Bundy, 2005), Nigeria (Ewu & Lakujo, 2005), and Scandinavia (Ilsaas & Kjølner, 2005).

Successful implementation of such artist-in-the-classroom initiatives hinges on twin factors that attitudinally reflect the degree to which arts are valued in schools, and practically reflect "the partnership between school officials and artist educators" (Pitter, 2005, p. 5). *Playlinks* offers evidence of both positive and negative facets of these two factors. Gattenhof (2001) identified two types of artist/school partnerships – instructional and administrative. Instructional partnership deals with actual work in the classroom, while administrative partnership is concerned with organizing, coordinating, governing, clarifying roles and responsibilities, and evaluating. *Playlinks* artists encountered various degrees of instructional partnership with teachers; Carousel Players' staff members maintained various degrees of administrative partnership with school principals.

My field notes attest that teacher involvement in *Playlinks* workshops varied greatly. Most observed as non-participants, a few directly interacted with students and the artist, some observed while engaged in other tasks, a few left the classroom for periods of time, and one texted on a cell phone throughout the workshop. One *Playlinks* actor commented:

> … some teachers were more engaged in the workshops than others. As a visitor to the classroom, sometimes I felt that the teacher was with me and we were working together …. Other times, I felt that the teacher completely disengaged and sat back and let me deliver the workshop. (Interview transcript, 5 June 2014)

Regarding administrative partnership, Carousel Players' staff worked diligently to communicate with principals about scheduling *Playlinks* workshops. In some schools, principals returned calls promptly and planned efficiently. In other schools, maintaining communication around scheduling dates and timetables was more troublesome. According to general manager, Jane Gardner:

> [A major problem was] communicating to principals and getting principals' buy-in …. Ensuring that they would actually book the pre-visit and the post-visit … in a timely way so they were close to the performance …. It's an amazing amount of time required, sometimes five to ten phone calls just to get a principal to fill out a piece of paper …. We

had to be very patient and organized and methodical to ensure that everything went smoothly. (Interview transcript, 6 June 2014)

In terms of valuing the arts, most *Playlinks* schools and teachers welcomed the opportunity for students to engage with professional actors as a beneficial learning resource. Some, however, appeared to view the workshops as either mere entertainment or practical convenience. In one school, for example, post-show workshops were deliberately scheduled on the school's pre-vacation "beach day", when children wore beach apparel to school and participated in "dance-offs" in the gymnasium. In another school, workshops were scheduled during a sports tournament that took several students away from class. It was not uncommon for workshops to be slated on days when teachers were attending professional development sessions, and classes were supervised by supply teachers who lacked awareness of the workshops until the artist arrived at the classroom door. Finally, two teachers I interviewed planned to use workshop activities to generate report card marks for drama. Their willingness to offer this information voluntarily in a recorded interview implies an inherent disrespect for the importance of drama as a required component of the Ontario curriculum.

According to one *Playlinks* actor:

> … some schools value the arts and that [respect] comes from the principal and the staff. Other schools see the arts as an "add-on" that's not essential … And I think those attitudes are the most difficult to battle because they filter down to the students. If the teacher and the principal view this workshop as kind of an interruption of their day or a little extra frivolous thing, then that's how the students view it. (Interview transcript, 5 June 2014)

Playlinks artists sometimes encountered multiple classes combined to receive the post-show workshop. My field notes documented that, although most students seemed highly involved in post-performance activities, a marked exception occurred in combined classes of Grades 7 and 8 (students aged 13–14 years), where several students appeared hesitant and inhibited. Actors commented on the hardship associated with large groups of students in a single session:

> …. often the groups were too big. [Some] principals seemed to want to put three classes together, which made it so much more difficult …. Then it becomes crowd management. You're not delivering an arts workshop anymore. You're just maintaining peace. You're maintaining some semblance of order in a large room. And it was very clear that those were the schools that didn't value what was being offered. (Interview transcript, 5 June 2014)
>
> I remember once there were about 60 students in one small classroom together …. That workshop was one of the most challenging just because there were so many people in the room. And I believe they were in first or second grade … Big groups in small spaces are really tough. (Interview transcript, 23 July 2014)

Teachers as well as artists commented on the ineffectiveness of combining classes for the workshops: "The group size of approximately 45 students was too busy. I would have liked a smaller group to explore more drama strategies" (Grade 3 teacher).

Despite obstacles encountered in both school attitudes towards drama and practicalities of scheduling, all stakeholders involved in *Playlinks* attested to its overall value. The reflective comments of two *Playlinks* actors offer an appropriate closing:

Playlinks was a wonderful way to scaffold [students'] understanding of theatre. And give them the opportunity to practice drama itself …. They got to see it, do it, understand it, and embody it. We took them through the whole process and that was really valuable. (Interview transcript, 5 June 2014)

I had some teachers say to me how great it was because their kids wouldn't otherwise get this sort of opportunity. These are kids who don't know that it's OK to be imaginative and creative without getting punished for it. These are kids who don't get to experience this. (Interview transcript, 23 July 2014)

Disclosure statement

No potential conflict of interest was reported by the author.

Funding

This work was supported by an Ontario Trillium Foundation Grant and the Social Sciences and Humanities Research Council of Canada [Grant number 430-2013-1025].

References

Andrews, B. W. (2010). Seeking harmony: Teachers' perspectives on learning to teach in and through the arts. *Encounters on Education, 11*, 81–98.

Bedard, R. (2011). Theatre for young audiences and cultural identity. In S. Schonmann (Ed.), *Key concepts in theatre/drama education* (pp. 283–287). Boston, MS: Sense Publishers.

Betts, J. D. (2005). Theatre arts integration at a middle school: Teacher professional development and drama experience. *Youth Theatre Journal, 19*, 17–33. doi:10.1080/08929092.2005.10012574

Bogdan, R., & Biklen, S. (1998). *Qualitative research for education* (3rd ed.). Toronto: Allyn and Bacon.

Bolton, G. (1984). *Drama as education: An argument for placing drama at the centre of the curriculum*. London: Longman.

Brinda, W., & Whordley, D. (2005). Bringing literature to life for reluctant and struggling adolescent readers with theatre for young audiences. *Stage of the Art, 17*(2), 15–17.

Brockett, O. G. (1985). Drama, a way of knowing. In J. H. Davis (Ed.), *Theatre education: Mandate for tomorrow* (pp. 1–5). New Orleans: Anchorage.

Bundy, P. (2003). Aesthetic engagement in process drama. *Research in Drama Education, 8*(2), 171–181. doi:10.1080/13569780308333

Cahill, H. (2014). Withholding the personal story: Using theory to orient practice in applied theatre about HIV and human rights. *Research in Drama Education, 19*(1), 23–38. doi:10.1080/13569783.2013.872427

Campbell, S., & Townshend, K. (1997). *Making the case for arts education.* Toronto: Ontario Arts Council.

Coopman, S. (1989). *Carousel Players: Participation theatre for young audiences.* Unpublished master's thesis. Guelph, ON: University of Guelph.

Craig, D., & Morgan, R. (1998). *Dib and Dob and the journey home.* Toronto, ON: Playwrights Guild of Canada.

Creswell, J. W. (2012). *Educational research* (4th ed.). Toronto, ON: Pearson.

Cusworth, R., & Simons, J. (1997). *Beyond the script: Drama in the classroom.* Sydney, Australia: PETA.

Duffy, P. (2014). The blended space between third and first person learning: Drama, cognition and transfer. *Research in Drama Education, 19*(1), 89–97. doi:10.1080/13569783.2013.872428

Eisner, E. W. (2005). The role of the arts in cognition and curriculum. In E. Eisner (Ed.ed.), *Reimagining schools [electronic resource]: The selected works of Elliot W. Eisner* (pp. 75-84)). London, UK: Taylor & Francis e-books, Routledge.

Ewu, J., & Lakujo, T. (2005). Unmasking the masquerades: The potential of TIE in Nigeria. In T. Jackson (Ed.), *Learning through theatre: New perspectives on theatre in education* (2nd ed., pp. 165–184). London, UK: Routledge.

Fairhead, W. (2005). Establishment or alternative: Two Canadian models. In T. Jackson (Ed.), *Learning through theatre: New perspectives on theatre in education* (2nd ed., pp. 151–164). London, UK: Routledge.

Gattenhof, S. (2001). More than just a handshake: Partnerships between artists and classrooms. *Drama Australia, 25*(2), 15–21.

Greene, M. (2011). Art and imagination: Overcoming a desperate stasis. In A. Ornstein, E. Pajak, & S. Ornstein (Eds.), *Contemporary issues in curriculum* (5th ed., pp. 33–40). Toronto, ON: Pearson.

Harvey, M., & Miles, D. (2009). And then they came for me: The effectiveness of a theatrical performance and study guide on middle-school students' holocaust knowledge and empathic concern. *Youth Theatre Journal, 23*(2), 91–102. doi:10.1080/08929090903281402

Horitz, T. (2006). Not our problem, is it? *Drama, 13*(2), 45–47.

Ilsaas, T., & Kjølner (2005). TIE in Scandanavia. In T. Jackson (Ed.), *Learning through theatre: New perspectives on theatre in education* (2nd ed., pp. 185–204). London, UK: Routledge.

Jackson, T. (2005). Introduction. In T. Jackson (Ed.), *Learning through theatre: New perspectives on theatre in education* (2nd ed., pp. 1–12). London, UK: Routledge.

Jackson, A. (2011). Participatory forms of educational theatre. In S. Schonmann (Ed.), *Key concepts in theatre/drama education* (pp. 289–293). Boston, MS: Sense Publishers.

Krathwohl, D., Bloom, B., & Masia, B. (1964). *Taxonomy of educational objectives: The classification of educational goals: Handbook II: Affective domain.* New York: McKay.

Klein, J. (2011). Criticism and appreciation in theatre for young audiences. In S. Schonmann (Ed.), *Key concepts in theatre/drama education* (pp. 235–240). Boston, MS: Sense Publishers.

Kvale, S., & Brinkmann, S. (2009). *Interviews: Learning the craft of qualitative research interviewing* (2nd ed.). Thousand Oaks, California: SAGE.

Lushington, K. (2003). The play's the thing: Lighting the fire of imagination through theatre and drama in Ontario schools. In *Professionally Speaking* (pp. 23–28). Toronto: Ontario College of Teachers..

McCaslin, N. (2006). *Creative drama in the classroom and beyond* (8th ed.). Boston: Pearson.

McLauchlan, D. (2001). Collaborative creativity in a high school drama class. *Youth Theatre Journal, 15*, 42–58. doi:10.1080/08929092.2001.10012530

McLauchlan, D. (2006). Teacher education in drama: Grooming lambs to meet wolves? In L. McCammon & D. McLauchlan (Eds.), *Universal mosaic of drama and theatre: The IDEA 2004 dialogues* (pp. 133–138). Queensland, Australia: IDEA Publications.

McLauchlan, D. (2009). Ontario teachers as target TYA audiences. *Youth Theatre Journal, 23*(2), 116–126. doi:10.1080/08929090903281428

Mertler, C. A., & Charles, C. M. (2005). *Introduction to educational research* (5th ed.). Toronto, ON: Pearson.

Miller, M. (1993/2013). *The power of Harriet T.* Toronto, ON: Theatre Fountainhead.

Neelands, J. (1990). *Structuring drama work.* New York, NY: Cambridge University Press.

Neuman, W. L. (2007). *Basics of social research* (2nd ed.). Toronto: Pearson.

Omasta, M. (2009). The TYA contract: A social contractarian approach to obligations between theatre for young audience (TYA) companies and their constituents. *Youth Theatre Journal, 23* (2), 103–115. doi:10.1080/08929090903281410

O'Toole, J., & Bundy, P. (2005). Kites and magpies: TIE in Australia. In T. Jackson (Ed.), *Learning through theatre: New perspectives on theatre in education* (2nd ed., pp. 133–150). London, UK: Routledge.

Patteson, A. (2005). *A summary of the program evaluation research, 1999-2005.* Toronto, ON: Learning through the Arts.

Pitter, J. (2005). *The arts ed "slim" kit: A resource for artists working in schools.* Toronto, ON: Ontario Arts Council.

Rabkin, N., & Redmond, R. (2006). The arts make a difference. *Educational Leadership, 63*(5), 60–64.

Riherd, M., & Hardwick, G. (2005). the creative arts team in the United States. In T. Jackson (Ed.), *Learning through theatre: New perspectives on theatre in education* (2nd ed., pp. 205–222). London, UK: Routledge.

Saldaña, J. (1995). "Is theatre necessary?": Final exit interviews with sixth grade participants from the ASU longitudinal study. *Youth Theatre Journal, 9,* 14–30. doi:10.1080/ 08929092.1995.10012462

Tooman, T. (2010). Affective learning: activities to promote values comprehension. *Soulstice training.* Retrieved from http://www.soulsticetraining.com/commentary/affective.html

Tuisku, H. V. (2015). Exploring bodily reactions: Embodied pedagogy as an alternative for conventional paradigms of acting in youth theatre education. *Youth Theatre Journal, 29*(1), 15–30. doi:10.1080/08929092.2015.1006713

Upitis, R., & Smithram, K. (2003). *National assessment 1999-2002. Final report to the Ontario Conservatory of Music.* Kingston, ON: Queen's University.

Walberg, H. T. (2011). Productive teachers: Assessing the knowledge base. In A. Ornstein, E. Pajak, & S. Ornstein (Eds.), *Contemporary issues in curriculum* (5th ed., pp. 94–109). Toronto, ON: Pearson.

Index